O P L

OXFORD PSYCHIATRY LIBRARY

Sleep Disorders

Second Edition

Dr Sue Wilson

Senior Research Fellow, Centre for Neuropsychopharmacology,
Division of Brain Sciences, Department of Medicine,
Imperial College London, London, UK

Prof. David J. Nutt

Professor of Neuropsychopharmacology,
Centre for Neuropsychopharmacology,
Division of Brain Sciences,
Department of Medicine, Imperial College London, London, UK

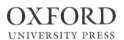

OXFORD
UNIVERSITY PRESS

OXFORD
UNIVERSITY PRESS

Great Clarendon Street, Oxford, OX2 6DP,
United Kingdom

Oxford University Press is a department of the University of Oxford.
It furthers the University's objective of excellence in research, scholarship,
and education by publishing worldwide. Oxford is a registered trade mark of
Oxford University Press in the UK and in certain other countries

First Edition published in 2008
Second Edition published in 2013

Impression: 4

Published in the United States of America by Oxford University Press
198 Madison Avenue, New York, NY 10016, United States of America

British Library Cataloguing in Publication Data
Data available

Library of Congress Control Number: 2013937233

ISBN 978–0–19–967455–8

Printed in the UK
by Ashford Colour Press Ltd., Gosport, Hampshire

Sleep Disorders

▶ Except where otherwise stated, drug doses and recommendations are for the non-pregnant adult who is not breast-feeding.

Contents

Preface to the first edition *vii*

Preface to the first edition

Sleep disorders are the orphans of medical practice, despite the fact that up to 40% of all primary care attendees have sleep symptoms, and in psychiatry practice this percentage rises; in depression almost everyone has a degree of sleep disturbance. In other psychiatric disorders the levels are lower but often highly important—for example, circadian disruption in schizophrenia and dementia severely impacts on rehabilitation possibilities, and insomnia in bipolar disorder is an early warning of manic relapse. Sleep is also important in other medical conditions, most notably sleep breathing disorders with their attendant daytime risks of sleepiness-induced accidents. Finally, there are some disorders of sleep itself, such as narcolepsy and night terrors, which though rare do have major impacts on the lives of patients and their relatives, as well as revealing insights into the brain mechanisms underlying sleep processes.

Despite this wide impact of disordered sleep in medical practice and the major impairments it causes to quality of life, most doctors and other health professionals have only minimal training in sleep processes or their pathology. This short book sets out to redress this imbalance by giving a concise yet complete overview of the field. We cover the basics of sleep physiology and then describe the wide range of different disorders that can be seen in both primary and secondary care. The ways to diagnose these are described, and treatment approaches are summarized. There is a special chapter dedicated to the problems of sleep disruption that we as professionals inevitably experience and often suffer from.

We believe that this book will fulfill a useful role in the education of doctors, nurses and other healthcare professionals. In addition, we hope that it will communicate some of our enthusiasm for this area of medicine in which we have worked for over 25 years.

David Nutt, March 2008

Chapter 1

Normal sleep

Key points

- Sleep is essential to normal brain function
- Loss of sleep can result in changes in mood, cognitive impairment, and abnormal hormone rhythms
- Most adults sleep for between 7 and 8 h a night; adults who sleep for less than 6 h are likely to report that they do not get enough sleep and that they are more dissatisfied with life
- The sleep–wake cycle is controlled by two separate but interacting processes: the *circadian* process and the *homeostatic* or *recovery* process
- The typical sleep pattern consists of 4 or 5 cycles of quiet sleep, alternating with paradoxical or rapid-eye-movement (REM) sleep
- Quiet sleep is often referred to as non-REM (NREM) sleep, and is divided further into four stages

1.1 Why do we sleep?

Humans spend about a third of their lives asleep, but we know surprisingly little about the precise function of sleep. What we do know is that:

- loss of sleep results in a wide variety of consequences, such as changes in mood, cognitive impairment, and abnormal hormone rhythms
- there is a rebound of sleep after a period of sleep deprivation, suggesting that its loss leads to a homeostatic compensatory increase.

From this, we can deduce that sleep is essential to brain function, and in support of this are very rare disorders such as fatal familial insomnia, in which almost total lack of sleep leads to an early death. Many research studies have shown that reductions in sleep are particularly impairing of learning and memory processes, and therefore sleep may be critical to neuronal plasticity.

1.2 How much sleep do we need?

Sleep is common to all animal species, but in only a few, notably primates, is there a single consolidated period of sleep once a day. Humans report varying times for their ideal period of sleep, but the majority of adults sleep for between 7 and 8 h a night.

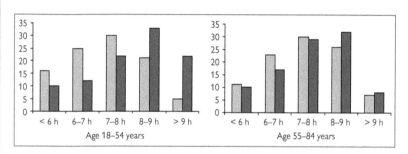

Figure 1.1 Hours of sleep reported on weekdays (light blue) and at weekends (darker blue). Based on data from the National Sleep Foundation (2002).

Those who habitually sleep for less than 6 h are likely to report that they sleep less than they would like to, and that they are more dissatisfied with life. People of school and working age, who have fixed morning start times, tend to sleep less during the week and 'catch up' at weekends.

The amount of sleep needed for each individual is simply the amount that is sufficient for them to be able to perform daytime activities satisfactorily and feel refreshed (see Figure 1.1).

1.3 How is sleep regulated?

Research over the past 25 years has proved that our sleep–wake cycle is controlled by two separate but interacting processes (Borbely 1982), namely the *circadian* process and the *homeostatic* or recovery process.

1.3.1 The circadian process

The circadian process is that which regulates the daily rhythms of the body and brain. Circadian (24-h) patterns of activity are found in many organs and even in individual cells. The main circadian pacemaker—our 'body clock'—is found in a group of cells in the suprachiasmatic nucleus (SCN) of the hypothalamus. These cells provide an oscillatory pattern of activity with a cycle time about every 24 h, which drives all of our bodily rhythms, including sleep–wake activity, hormone release, liver function, etc.

- This drive from the SCN is innate, self-sustaining, and independent of tiredness or amount of sleep.
- It is affected markedly by light and to some extent by temperature.
- Bright light in the evening will delay the clock and bright light in the morning is necessary to synchronize the clock to a 24-h rhythm.
- In constant light or darkness, the cycle length is about 24.3 h.

In fact, the light cycle that is determined by the earth's rotation effectively shortens the SCN cycle and keeps it to 24 h. Light is therefore called a zeitgeber (timekeeper) of circadian rhythms.

All animals have these clocks, and their period and timing appear to be dependent on particular genes, most of which are common to fruit flies, mice, and primates, and probably many other species. Mutations (polymorphisms) of these genes that lead to an altered circadian rhythm are particularly easy to identify in fruit flies, and similar variants of these genes have been found in people with certain disorders of circadian rhythm. Particular disorders of sleep scheduling—for example, delayed sleep phase disorder (see Chapter 6)—have been shown to have a high association with a particular form of a clock gene (Ebisawa 2007).

It seems that both how long we sleep and our preferred sleep timing (whether or not we are evening people or 'owls', or morning people or 'larks') is partly dependent on our genetic makeup. The molecular processes whereby genes interact with brain mechanisms, making the clock 'tick', have been well worked out and involve the production of proteins that activate cell metabolism, which then silences the genes responsible for their own production over a 24-h cycle (see Vitaterna *et al* 2001).

The drive to sleep from the circadian clock (called the 'C' process) starts slowly at around 11 p.m. and gradually increases to peak at about 4 a.m. (see Figure 1.2). The clock provides a sleep-promoting process, which continues into mid-morning and then provides a wakefulness-promoting process during the day.

1.3.2 The homeostatic process

The *homeostatic* or recovery drive to sleep (called the 'S' process) is wake-dependent—that is, it increases in proportion to the amount of time the person has been awake since their last sleep. It usually reaches a maximum at about 11 p.m., or about 16 h after waking up in the morning, and it then decreases during sleep, with a minimum at natural waking in the morning. When sleep has been shorter than usual, there is a 'sleep debt', which leads to an increase in the S process—this works to ensure that the debt is made up at the next sleep period by accelerating the time to sleep and possibly by increasing sleep depth and duration.

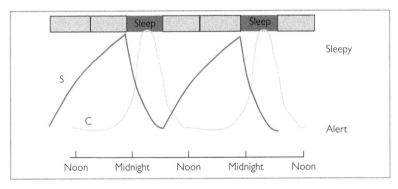

Figure 1.2 The two sleep processes. The light blue line, C, is the circadian sleep propensity, which reaches a maximum at around 4 a.m. and tails off during the morning, keeping us alert during the day and early evening. The darker blue line is the homeostatic sleep process S, which reaches a maximum after about 16 h of being awake and rapidly declines during sleep.

These two processes interact to promote the onset of sleep when both are high (at the usual bedtime), and to maintain sleep when the C process is high and the S process is declining (in the small hours).

There is also an increase in circadian sleep propensity in the afternoon. In those societies where a biphasic sleep pattern is—or at least was—common, such as those around the Mediterranean, the siesta is taken at around 2–4 p.m. This afternoon sleep satisfies the S process, which is then low again until much later in the day. This explains why the second sleep period (at night) can be delayed until 1 or 2 a.m. The afternoon increase in sleep propensity is often called the 'post-lunch dip', but no lunch needs to be eaten for us to experience it—it is just a clock phenomenon. There is also a period of increased drive to be awake in mid-evening, when physical and intellectual functioning is high, and it is difficult to fall asleep. This is often called the 'forbidden zone' for sleep, and is the reason why going to sleep early is so much more difficult than sleeping on in the morning.

1.3.3 Arousal, relaxation, and anxiety

The process of being aroused or alert may overcome either of these previous sleep-promoting processes, and is one of the main mechanisms involved in insomnia. If mentally, emotionally, or physically arousing activities take place near our expected sleeping time, then the time to fall asleep will be longer than usual. These arousal-producing activities can include studying, watching a very disturbing movie, having an argument, or just worrying, as well as exercising or otherwise physically exerting oneself. Sex seems to be an exception, perhaps because hormones or other chemicals such as prostaglandins are released during and after sex, and some of these, such as oxytocin, may be sleep promoting, presumably to encourage rest to facilitate sperm progress to fertilization of the egg.

In the daytime, boredom and inactivity can reduce arousal and cause sleepiness, which overcomes the circadian and homeostatic drives to be awake.

1.4 Physiology of sleep–wake control

There has been an explosion of recent studies of the physiology of sleep–wake regulation as new research technology has become available. The peptide orexin (hypocretin) has been found to be crucial for regulating wakefulness and hence sleep (for a review, see Kukkonen 2013). These studies show that sleep and wakefulness are regulated by groups of neurons whose cell bodies are located in the hypothalamus and brainstem and whose activity stabilizes the behavioural state of either sleep or wakefulness and allows fast switching between sleep and wakefulness.

During wakefulness, the ascending arousal system is predominant, and during sleep this is inhibited by sleep-controlling neurons (see Chapter 9).

1.5 Structure of sleep

Sleep is a state of physical inactivity accompanied by loss of awareness and a markedly reduced responsiveness to environmental stimuli. Recording the EEG and other physiological variables such as muscle activity and eye movements during sleep (a

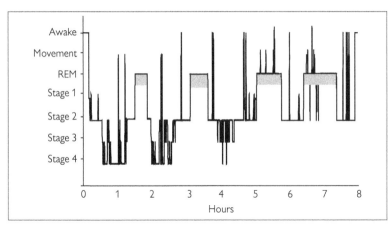

Figure 1.3 A normal hypnogram, showing the stages of sleep and their distribution over the night.

technique called polysomnography) gives information about the different stages of sleep and their pattern of occurrence. This pattern varies from person to person, but usually consists of four or five cycles of quiet sleep alternating with paradoxical and rapid-eye-movement (REM) sleep. The first part of the night is characterized by periods of deep quiet sleep with more and longer periods of REM sleep in the latter half of the night. A representation of these various stages over time is known as a hypnogram, and one of these derived from a normal subject is shown in Figure 1.3.

The quiet sleep is often referred to as non-REM (NREM), and is divided further into four stages. Stage 1 ('dozing') is a very light sleep halfway between sleep and waking, when most people would say they were just 'resting their eyes' if it happened during the day. Stage 2 is slightly deeper, sometimes with occasional small jerks, and relaxed muscles and slightly slower breathing and heart rate than during waking. When woken from this stage, about 50% of people would say that they had been asleep. When someone is in deep sleep, stages 3 and 4, they look pale and peaceful and the heart rate and breathing are slowed. It is difficult to wake them up, and they are disorientated on waking, sometimes for up to 10 min. Progression between these four stages is gradual and characterized in the electroencephalogram (EEG) by increasing amounts of slow synchronous activity as the arousal of cortex is decreased and the cortex and thalamus show increased synchrony of firing rates. Stages 3 and 4 sleep are known as slow-wave sleep (SWS), because high-amplitude slow (delta) waves predominate (see Table 1.1). In this deep sleep, restorative processes in the body take place; for instance, growth hormone is released mainly during slow-wave sleep.

In contrast, the entry into REM sleep is rapid and fairly sudden. During REM sleep, the EEG appearance is similar to that of waking or stage 1 sleep, implying that the cortex is active (this gave rise to the term 'paradoxical' sleep), and there are frequent jerky movements of the eyes (the rapid eye movements after which it is now named). However, the main difference compared with the awake state is that, during REM, there is complete paralysis of the skeletal muscles—the person is in effect paralysed—presumably

Stage of sleep	EEG features	Eye movements	EMG activity
Waking	Low-amplitude, mixed, and sometimes alpha rhythm	Many, varied, usually fast	High
1	Low-amplitude, mainly irregular theta activity, and triangular vertex waves	Slow, rolling lateral movements	Slightly lowered
2	Sleep spindles, K complexes, and some low-amplitude theta and delta activity	None	Lowered
3	High-amplitude delta activity for 20–50% of the time, spindles less prominent, and K complexes longer, and less discrete	None	Low
4	Same as 3, with delta activity for >50% of the time	None	Low
REM	Low-amplitude, irregular mixed activity, and sometimes saw-toothed waves	Rapid, jerky, and usually lateral movements in clusters	Virtually absent, occasional short bursts

Table 1.1 EEG, eye movement, and muscle features associated with the stages of sleep

to prevent them acting out their dreams and to provide optimal rest for restoration of muscle function. This paralysis is demonstrated by the loss of activity on the electromyogram (EMG), which is usually recorded from the muscles under the chin. In rare cases, muscle paralysis during sleep is not complete, and problems such as REM behaviour disorder appear (see Chapter 5). During REM, there is an increase in autonomic arousal relative to that in the other sleep stages, with irregular breathing. REM is the sleep stage when most dreaming takes place.

As can be seen from the hypnogram, a normal subject will have several short awakenings during the night, most of which are not perceived as awakenings unless they last more than about 2 min. Probably there will not be clear consciousness, but there may be an occasional brief thought about how comfortable the subject is or how pleased they are that it is not time to get up yet, followed by an immediate return to sleep. If during the short period of waking there is some factor that causes anger or anxiety, such as aircraft noise, a partner's snoring, or anxiety about being awake, the awakening is more likely to be remembered. Checking the time (clock-watching) often leads to irritation and arousal, which can then impair the person's ability to get back to sleep and lead to dissatisfaction with sleep quality.

1.5.1 EEG phenomena during sleep

Slow-wave (delta) activity is defined as having a frequency of between 0.5 and 4 Hz. It is not present during the daytime in a normal adult EEG, but it is present during sleep (and also to a greater degree in coma). Slow-wave activity is recorded at maximal amplitude over the frontal lobes, but is widespread across the brain. It gradually increases in amplitude and becomes more synchronous as sleep becomes deeper, a process thought to be generated in the thalamocortical loop system. SWS can therefore be thought of as

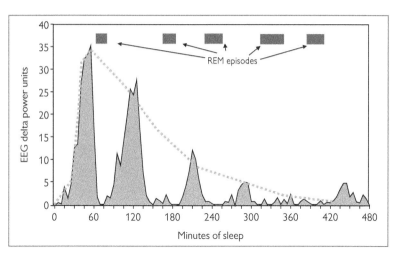

Figure 1.4 Pattern of electroencephalogram (EEG) slow waves during the night. Most occur during the first cycle of sleep, and they gradually diminish over the course of the night (dotted line).

an 'idling' process when the upward arousal system from the brainstem via the thalamus to the cortex is inactive. This is borne out by evidence from positron emission tomography (PET) and functional magnetic resonance imaging (fMRI) which suggests that metabolism and blood flow are reduced in the cortex during SWS.

The EEG slow waves are more obvious and of higher amplitude during the first cycle of sleep and gradually diminish during the night, following the same pattern as the sleep drive from the homeostatic process (see Figure 1.4). In fact, slow or delta activity is a marker of the homeostatic role of sleep, because following sleep deprivation, slow waves show a marked rebound in amount, amplitude, and synchronicity in recovery sleep. This rebound in slow waves is proportional to the sleep loss. Thus if we lose a night's sleep, this homeostatic drive is paramount, and we will have twice the usual amount of SWS the following night.

K complexes and sleep spindles are phenomena of sleep that are routinely used to score sleep stages, and are related to the transmission of information from the thalamus to the cortex. K complexes can be evoked readily in light sleep by auditory stimulation, and it is thought that these are manifestations of a downward signal (from the cortex to the thalamus and brainstem) to stay asleep. Sleep spindles are short bursts of rhythmic 10–15 Hz activity which occur during light and deep non-REM sleep, and may be related to preventing the cortex from processing during sleep.

1.6 Sleep in special populations

1.6.1 Sleep in children

Sleep changes markedly over the first few years of life. The 24-h rhythm does not develop immediately, but gradually becomes apparent over the first 3 months of life.

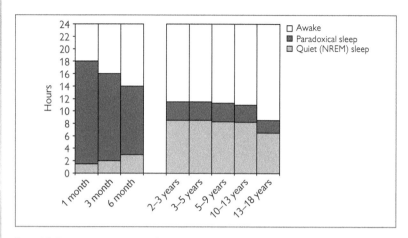

Figure 1.5 Approximate proportions of waking and sleep in children. Figure 1.5 is based on data from Dittrichova J (1966). Development of sleep in infancy. *J Appl Physiol* **21**:1243–6, and Roffwarg HP, Muzio JN, Dement WC (1966). Ontogenetic development of the human sleep-dream cycle. *Science* **152**: 604–19.

However, some elements of a 24-h cycle are apparent very early on. Babies seem to have got the hang of the evening 'forbidden zone' by 2–3 weeks of age and are less likely to sleep in the evening, as any parent knows.

The structure of sleep also changes greatly in childhood. Sleep features are different from those in adults, and scoring of sleep into stages is more difficult. However, quiet sleep (called NREM in adults) and paradoxical active sleep are apparent from birth, although the accompanying eye movements are not obvious in early infancy. Paradoxical sleep predominates in very young infants and gradually decreases over the course of childhood and adolescence. Deep slow-wave sleep occurs during a large part of the night that is not occupied by REM sleep. This predominance of deep sleep gradually diminishes from the teenage years onward, with more light sleep taking its place (see Figure 1.5).

1.6.2 **Sleep and ageing**

During adult life there are two major changes in sleep. First, the amount of time awake in bed increases as we get older, mostly due to increased fragmentation of sleep. Secondly, the amount of slow-wave sleep decreases and, along with this, growth hormone secretion also falls. Figure 1.6 shows some findings from a series of important studies (Van Cauter *et al* 2000) that describe the changes in sleep and hormones in a cohort of 149 healthy men.

1.6.3 **Sleep during pregnancy and menopause**

Epidemiological studies clearly indicate changes in women's sleep quality in association with alterations in hormonal levels during pregnancy and menopause. Many women complain of poor sleep during pregnancy. In the first trimester, nausea, backache, and urinary frequency can cause sleep disturbance. The second trimester tends to be easier,

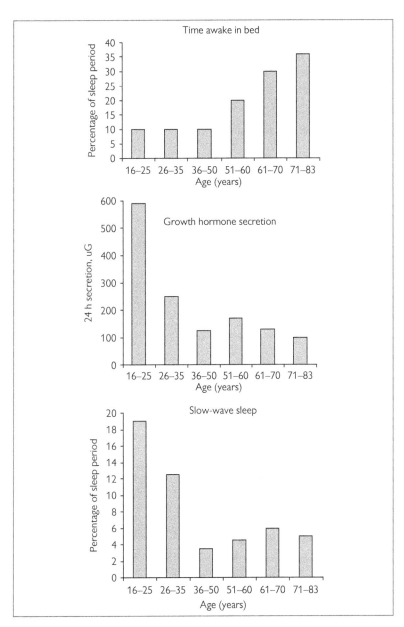

Figure 1.6 Change in waking time, slow-wave sleep, and growth hormone secretion with age in adult men. Based on data from Van Cauter et al (2000).

but fetal movements and heartburn may be problematic. By the third trimester, sleep is more disturbed, with complaints of urinary frequency and backache again, in addition to cramps, itch, and unpleasant dreams. Most women fall asleep easily but wake more frequently.

A US study of normal sleepers showed that women sleep more deeply than men, and that the menopause is associated with longer sleep latency and decreased slow-wave sleep. In addition, it was found that hormone therapy appeared to protect women from these unfavourable changes (Bixler et al 2009). The incidence of sleep disorders is also affected by gender and hormone status (see Chapters 4 and 8).

1.7 Sleep and dreaming

Discussion of the content and meaning of dreams is beyond the scope of this book, but the processes underlying this fascinating phenomenon are becoming better understood. Nearly everyone dreams, but dreams are usually only remembered when there is a period of waking during or at the end of a REM episode. Dreams can occur during NREM sleep, too, although these dreams may be generally different—they are less story-like and bizarre. Eye movements and twitching during REM sleep occur in bouts lasting from seconds to 2–3 min (called 'phasic' REM), alternating with periods of no movement lasting for 1–3 min. It is plausible to suppose that these eye movements seen in REM sleep involve scanning of dream images, but this is hard to prove, because when subjects are woken during a bout of REM, the recall could be related to either of these types of REM. Nightmares are dreams that have an unpleasant or scary content that often leads to such high levels of arousal that the dreamer awakes in fear and so remembers the content as a nightmare. Although nightmares are experienced by most people at some stage in their life, they are more common in those with other psychiatric disorders, especially depression (see Chapter 7).

1.8 Sleep, learning, and memory

The influence of sleep on learning and memory is a controversial subject, but one of growing interest. There has been a huge increase in studies of memory consolidation and its relationship to sleep over the past few years. An improvement of performance on several tasks involving memory consolidation and procedural learning after sleep has been clearly shown, and the improvements seen after sleep are generally greater than those found after a period of rest without sleep, suggesting a special influence of sleep on learning. It is now widely accepted that sleep facilitates not only the storage of newly acquired notions and skills, but also their integration with pre-existing ones, However, the type, duration, and features of sleep, and the brain circuits involved, are complex, and new information is emerging daily (Conte and Ficca 2013). Many aspects of sleep are involved (e.g. both REM and non-REM sleep), and the role of particular sleep features, such as sleep spindles, in the study of these learning and memory processes is becoming clearer. For instance, we now know that the number and type of sleep spindles is related to learning ability, that they increase when learning has taken place during the preceding day, that this increase is related to sleep-dependent improvement in the learning task, and that they may reflect efficient thalamocortical communication (Fogel and Smith 2011).

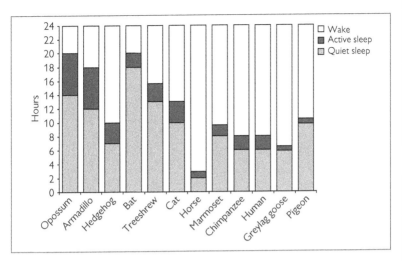

Figure 1.7 Sleeping and waking times of a range of animal species during a 24-h period. Based on data from Lesku *et al* (2006, and Roth *et al* (2006)).

1.9 Sleep in animals

All animals sleep, and mammals and birds have both quiet slow-wave and active para-doxical sleep, although not all move their eyes during the latter, and it is characterized by the loss of muscle tone and twitches. One thing that distinguishes the primates is the monophasic nature of their sleep—that is, they have most of their sleep in one period. This can be at night or during daylight. For instance, humans and some primates, horses, and cows have all their sleep in the hours of darkness, whereas rats and mice have only 30–40% of their sleep in darkness, and cats have 50%. Another difference is the consolidation of sleep periods. Different animals have different amounts of sleep taken during one episode; these vary from humans, whose sleep is 100% consolidated, to guinea pigs, which have most of their sleep in tiny bouts scattered throughout the day.

For those interested in the sleep habits of animals, the sleeping and waking times of a range of species are shown in Figure 1.7, taken from data provided by Lesku *et al* (2006, 2008).

References

Bixler EO, Papaliaga MN, Vgontzas AN *et al* (2009). Women sleep objectively better than men and the sleep of young women is more resilient to external stressors: effects of age and meno-pause. *J Sleep Res* **18**: 221–8.

Borbely AA (1982). A two-process model of sleep regulation. *Hum Neurobiol* **1**: 195–204.

Conte F, Ficca G (2013). Caveats on psychological models of sleep and memory: a compass in an overgrown scenario. *Sleep Med Rev* **17**: 105–21.

Dittrichova J (1966). Development of sleep in infancy. *J Appl Physiol* **21**: 1243–6.

Ebisawa T (2007). Circadian rhythms in the CNS and peripheral clock disorders: human sleep disorders and clock genes. *J Pharmacol Sci* **103**: 150–54.

Fogel SM, Smith CT (2011). The function of the sleep spindle: a physiological index of intelligence and a mechanism for sleep-dependent memory consolidation. *Neurosci Biobehav Rev* **35**: 1154–65.

Kukkonen JP (2013). Physiology of the orexinergic/hypocretinergic system: a revisit in 2012. *Am J Physiol Cell Physiol* **304**: C2–32.

Lesku JA, Roth TC, Amlaner CJ, Lima SL (2006). A phylogenetic analysis of sleep architecture in mammals: the integration of anatomy, physiology, and ecology. *Am Nat* **168**: 441–53.

Lesku JA, Roth TC, Rattenborg NC, Amlaner CJ, Lima SL (2008). Phylogenetics and the correlates of mammalian sleep: a reappraisal. *Sleep Med Rev* **12**: 229–44.

National Sleep Foundation (2002). *2002 'Sleep in America' Poll.* <www.sleepfoundation.org/sites/default/files/2002SleepInAmericaPoll.pdf>

Roffwarg HP, Muzio JN, Dement WC (1966). Ontogenetic development of the human sleep-dream cycle. *Science* **152**: 604–19.

Roth TC 2nd, Lesku JA, Amlaner CJ, Lima SL (2006). A phylogenetic analysis of the correlates of sleep in birds. *J Sleep Res* **15**: 395–402.

Van Cauter CE, Leproult R, Plat L (2000). Age-related changes in slow wave sleep and REM sleep and relationship with growth hormone and cortisol levels in healthy men. *JAMA* **284**: 861–8.

Vitaterna MH, Takahashi JS, Turek FW (2001). Overview of circadian rhythms. *Alcohol Res Health* **25**: 85–93

Chapter 2

Diagnosing sleep disorders

Key points

- Obtaining a sleep history is a critical part of the general examination of a patient presenting with a sleep disorder
- Sleep disorders are formally classified in both *ICD-10* and the *Diagnostic and Statistical Manual IV (DSM-IV)*, and are more fully described in the *International Classification of Sleep Disorders*
- Sleep disorders can be divided by symptom presentation into three major categories: insomnias, hypersomnias, and parasomnias
- Common precipitating factors of disordered sleep include irregular routine, caffeine, cigarettes, and alcohol and other drugs
- Questionnaires and sleep diaries can be helpful to the clinician in establishing a sleep diagnosis
- Specialist sleep centres have facilities for performing a range of objective tests of sleep and sleepiness, including actigraphy, polysomnography, multiple sleep latency testing, and overnight video recording

13

Taking a sleep history is a critical part of the general history and examination of a patient with a sleep disorder. In fact, asking the question 'How is your sleep at the moment?' should be part of a standard medical consultation, because sleep disorders are associated with a wide range of psychiatric and medical disorders.

The patient may indicate that they themselves have a problem with sleep or that their bed partner is worried about their night-time behaviour. Where possible, a consultation with the partner should be carried out, as it can throw much light on the nature of the sleep complaint and the issues that may be causing it.

Sleep disorders are formally classified in both standard diagnostic manuals, and are more fully described in the International Classification of Sleep Disorders. A very simplified symptom-led classification can be summarized as follows:

- insomnia—not enough sleep, or sleep of poor quality
- hypersomnia—excessive daytime sleepiness
- parasomnia—unusual happenings in the night.

The symptoms may point to one of these groups, but there are some disorders that may cause more than one group of symptoms.

Insomnia itself is often divided into three subtypes:

- onset insomnia—difficulty getting off to sleep
- maintenance insomnia—waking repeatedly in the night
- early-morning insomnia—waking too early and not being able to get back to sleep.

2.1 Ask 'What is the problem with sleep?'

Patients are very often vague at first about the nature of their complaint, saying 'My sleep is getting me down', 'I have terrible sleep', or 'My sleep pattern is all over the place', or just stating that they think they have insomnia. Some preliminary questions can be asked to give an indication of the symptoms they may have.

2.2 Symptoms at presentation

Useful questions about insomnia include the following:

- How long does it take you to get off to sleep? Do you wake up a lot during the night? Does it take you a long time to get back to sleep? How would you describe the quality of your sleep? Do you feel refreshed in the morning?
- How many 'bad' nights do you have in a week? What impact does this have on your daytime activities?

Useful questions about other sleep disorders include the following:

- Do you feel sleepy or take naps during the day (hypersomnia or poor sleep habits)?
- How has your mood been recently? Do you manage to enjoy your social/family activities (depression)?
- Do you find you cannot keep still at night? Do your legs twitch in bed (restless leg syndrome, RLS; periodic leg movements in sleep, PMLS)?
- Have you been told that you act strangely during your sleep (parasomnias)?
- Do you fall asleep suddenly during the day? Do you sometimes become weak when you are emotionally aroused—for instance, when you are laughing (narcolepsy)?
- Have you been told that you snore loudly? Have you been told that you stop breathing at night (obstructive sleep apnoea syndrome, OSAS)?

These questions should provide a starting point for exploring the problem. They should be followed by questions about symptom frequency, duration, severity, and impact on health and quality of life, treatments already tried, and whether or not those treatments worked. The partner's perception of the problem should be documented. Other useful information can include a history of sleep disorders in childhood or in other members of the family, and any medication that the person is taking, as many prescription drugs can affect sleep.

2.3 Further questions

It is important to ask about possible common precipitating factors, such as employment, caffeine, cigarettes, alcohol, and other drugs.

Employment-related stress is a common contributing factor in poor sleep; a typical pattern is 'Sunday-night insomnia' caused by worry about going to work the next day. Some jobs interfere with sleep—for example, those that require being on overnight call (e.g. doctors and nurses; see Chapter 10) and those that involve shift work. Losing a job—as with losing any important relationship, such as occurs in bereavement—is often associated with poor sleep accompanied by dreams and nightmares and onset insomnia.

Drugs can increase arousal and impair sleep. These include *caffeine* and theophylline/theobromine-containing drinks such as tea, coffee, and cola, as well as other stimulants such as nicotine and amphetamines. Sometimes these actions may be beneficial—for example, caffeine can reduce the risk of falling asleep when driving, and so is a recommended driving safety measure. Other drugs may initially promote sleep, but adaptive changes in the brain can then lead to insomnia in withdrawal. The most common of these is of course *alcohol*, which many people use in the form of a 'nightcap' to promote sleep. However, when taken in moderation, alcohol is cleared by the liver quite quickly and so can lead to a degree of morning withdrawal that often disrupts sleep. Long-term sleep disruption is also seen during *withdrawal* from drugs, especially benzodiazepines, barbiturates, cannabis, and opiates.

2.4 **Diagnosing insomnia**

The diagnosis of insomnia requires a report of consistently poor sleep, with difficulty either in getting off to sleep or in maintaining sleep, together with the complaint of impaired daytime function as a result of poor sleep. The patient's sleep habits, including appropriate scheduling of regular and adequate sleep times, and attention to intake of sleep-disturbing substances, should be satisfactory. Once this has been established and other disorders have been eliminated as described above, the diagnosis may be made (see Figure 2.1).

2.5 **Questionnaires**

A useful questionnaire, which patients can fill out in the waiting room, is the Bristol Sleep Profile (Smith *et al* 2001). This provides a basis for more in-depth questioning about lifestyle and specific sleep disorders.

A sleep diary is almost essential when exploring sleep problems. For instance, insomnia symptoms are rarely exactly the same from night to night, and a 2- or 3-week diary will provide information about the regularity and timing of sleep patterns and the frequency of symptoms.

The sleep diary in Table 2.1 reveals that the patient's preferred sleeping time at weekends is later than that in the week, which may indicate a sleep-scheduling disorder. An extra column to record medications can be added if required.

Questionnaires that are mainly research-oriented but which may be helpful in clinical use are the Pittsburgh Sleep Quality Index, which asks about sleep during the previous month (Buysse *et al* 1989), and the St Mary's Sleep Questionnaire (Ellis *et al* 1981) and the Leeds Sleep Evaluation Questionnaire (Parrott and Hindmarch 1978), which describe sleep on the previous night.

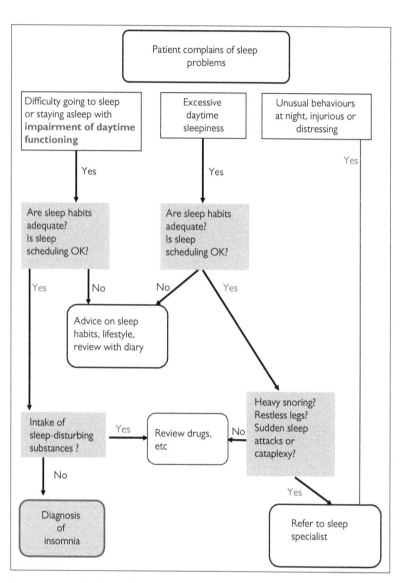

Figure 2.1 An algorithm for initial diagnosis of sleep disorders from the British Association for Psychopharmacology consensus statement on evidence-based treatment of insomnia, parasomnias and circadian rhythm disorders. Wilson SJ, Nutt DJ, Alford C et al. *J Psychopharmacol* **24**: 1577–601, © 2010 by British Association for Psychopharmacology. Reprinted by permission of SAGE.

Table 2.1 Extract from sleep diary

Name

Day	Time you went to bed last night	Time you fell asleep (roughly)	Time you finally woke up this morning (tick if the alarm woke you)	Time you got up	Number of times you woke up in the night	How many hours sleep you got overall	Quality of sleep (out of 10, from 1 = very bad to 10 = very good)	Comment (can include morning feeling, medication taken, etc)
Wednesday 7 June	2 a.m.	3 a.m.	9.30 a.m.	10.30 a.m.	1	6 h	6	Off work
Thursday 8 June	11.15 p.m.	1.30 a.m.	7 a.m. ✓	7 a.m.	4	3 h	3	Felt sleepy
Friday 9 June	11.30 p.m.	1 a.m.	7 a.m. ✓	7 a.m.	2	4 h	4	
Saturday 10 June	2 a.m.	3 a.m.	9 a.m.	9.30 a.m.	1	6 h	6	
Sunday 11 June	3 a.m.	3.30 a.m.	10 a.m.	10 a.m.	2	6 h	6	
Monday 12 June	11 p.m.	3 a.m.	7 a.m. ✓	7 a.m.	4	3 h	2	Felt lousy this morning
Tuesday 13 June	10.30 p.m.	2 a.m.	7 a.m. ✓	7 a.m.	2	3 h	2	Tired

Box 2.1 **Epworth Sleepiness Scale**

How likely are you to doze off or fall asleep in the following situations, in contrast to just feeling tired? This refers to your usual way of life in recent times. Even if you have not done some of these things recently, try to work out how they would have affected you. Use the following scale to choose the most appropriate number for each situation:

0 = no chance of dozing
1 = slight chance of dozing
2 = moderate chance of dozing
3 = high chance of dozing

SITUATION   SCORE

Sitting and reading. . . . .

Watching TV. . . . .

Sitting inactive in a public place (e.g. a theatre or a meeting) . . . .

As a passenger in a car for an hour without a break . . . .

Lying down to rest in the afternoon when circumstances permit . . . .

Sitting and talking to someone . . . .

Sitting quietly after a lunch without alcohol . . . .

In a car, while stopped for a few minutes in traffic. . . . .

TOTAL . . . .

If the patient says that they are tired during the day, it is important to establish whether or not this means actual sleepiness or fatigue. A useful quick questionnaire for this is the Epworth Sleepiness Questionnaire (Johns 1991) (see Box 2.1), which asks about the likelihood of actually falling asleep in common situations. Insomniacs in general have difficulty falling asleep at any time, so if there is a high score on the Epworth scale, then hypersomnia is more likely.

Scoring more than 10 on this scale should raise suspicion of a problem, and scoring more than 15 denotes pathological sleepiness.

2.6 **Objective tests**

Specialist sleep centres have facilities for performing a range of objective tests of sleep and sleepiness. They are described in the section that follows, and in later chapters there is a description of the situations in which they might be used as diagnostic aids.

2.6.1 **Actigraphy**

Actigraphy is a method of monitoring movement over days or weeks in real-life situations. It utilizes a small wrist-worn monitor containing a solid-state device (accelerometer) that produces electrical impulses in response to movements, which are stored in a digital memory (see Figure 2.2). Usually an actigraph records both intensity and duration of movements. It is light and easy to wear and can be used in non-compliant subjects (e.g. infants, patients with dementia). The actigraph gives a recording of rest

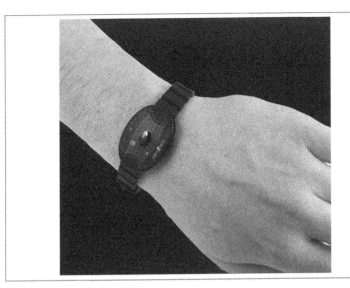

Figure 2.2 An actigraph monitor, which measures and records movement over a period of weeks.

and activity over a period of weeks and can be downloaded quickly to give an instant picture when the patient comes to clinic (see Figures 2.3 and 2.4).

Actigraphy may be useful for quantifying sleep as long as *wakefulness is associated with moving* and *sleep is associated with being still*. Thus the patient who lies still but awake in bed will be assumed to be asleep when the software sleep analysis is used, and people who are very restless during sleep will be assumed to have awoken, even if they have not. Actigraphy is best accompanied by some kind of daily log or diary so that unusual patterns may be seen in context.

2.6.2 Polysomnography (PSG)

Although actigraphy is relatively cheap and quite convenient, it provides no information about what is going on in the brain overnight or the physiological changes that occur during sleep. Overnight polysomnography (PSG) (which means the measurement of several physiological sleep variables) is the only way of providing this information. It involves attaching recording electrodes to the scalp, forehead, and chin to record electroencephalogram (EEG) eye movements or electro-oculogram (EOG) and muscle activity from the submental muscle (electromyogram, EMG). In addition, variables such as electrocardiogram (ECG), EMG from leg muscles, a range of respiratory variables, and body movements may be measured at the same time. Guidelines for minimal recording standards and for staging sleep were laid down by an international committee in the 1960s (Rechtschaffen and Kales 1968). In most sleep centres, PSG involves overnight admission to a sleep clinic, but some centres perform the investigations in the patient's home using battery-powered portable recording devices that are about the size of a portable hard disc (see Figure 2.5).

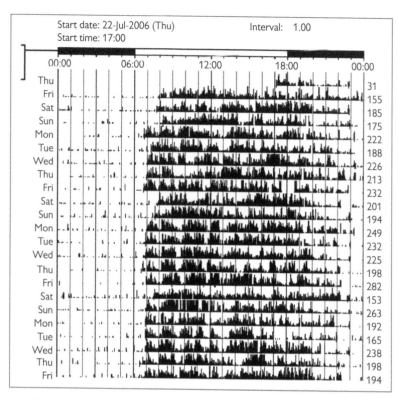

Figure 2.3 A typical actigraphy display. Each horizontal line represents one 24-h period, and vertical lines represent the sum of activity for each 1 min of that day. This example shows someone with a very regular lifestyle. Activity is markedly reduced from about 11 p.m. each day (when they go to bed) until about 7 a.m. on weekdays and 7–8 a.m. at weekends (when they get up); in between these two times we assume the subject is asleep. There is lower activity in the evening when the subject's activities were watching TV or gardening.

Information is recorded and then played back offline so that waveforms may be interpreted and sleep for each 30 s of the night scored for sleep stages (see Chapter 1).

Many other variables that can be derived are mentioned in reports from sleep centres and in research studies, and it may be useful to know what they mean.

Terms used in polysomnography reports include the following:

- time in bed (TIB)—this may mean actual time in bed, but it often means time from when the subject first closed their eyes until the time they woke in the morning
- sleep onset—usually to established (i.e. stage 2 of more than 1 min) sleep
- sleep onset latency (SOL)—time from either lights out or eyes closed to sleep onset

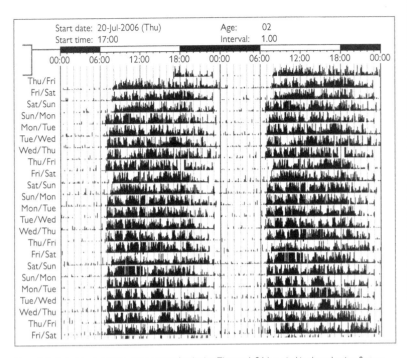

Figure 2.4 A double plot of the same actigraphy display. Thus each 24-h period is plotted twice, first on the right and then on the line below on the left. This kind of plot is useful for showing shifts of sleep–wake pattern in disruptions of circadian rhythm.

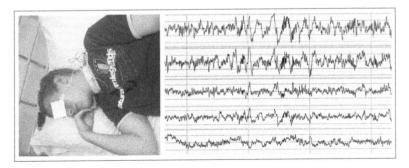

Figure 2.5 A subject demonstrating the size of an ambulatory overnight sleep recording device (just next to the head) with the neck collar supporting the connections from the scalp and eye and chin connections. On the right are some waveforms from a 20 s section of the recording.

- sleep period—time from sleep onset to end of sleep
- total sleep time—sum of time in each stage of sleep
- number of awakenings—depending on local conventions, these may have to be for as little as 30 s up to 2 min
- sleep efficiency—this usually means total sleep time as a percentage of time in bed, but it can mean as a percentage of sleep period (the latter excludes sleep onset latency)
- wake after sleep onset—total time awake during sleep period
- REM onset latency—time to beginning of first REM period of more than 1 min
- time in each sleep stage (total and sometimes separately for the first and second halves of the night)
- sleep stages as a percentage of total sleep time.

Variables related to respiration which are generally reported are the apnoea–hypopnoea index, which describes the number of breathing pauses per hour, and the desaturation index, which describes the number of times the patient's oxygen saturation (as measured by finger or earlobe oximetry) drops by (usually) 4% per hour or for the whole night.

Movements of the legs are rated if there is a question of PLMS, and these are described by an index of number of leg movements per hour (PLMS Index).

2.6.3 **Multiple Sleep Latency Test (MSLT)**

This is a standardized method for objectively assessing a person's propensity to sleep in the daytime, and thus for helping to diagnose or exclude the diagnosis of disorders such as excessive daytime sleepiness or narcolepsy. It must be performed after an overnight sleep recording, to check that night-time sleep has been as usual, and it is usually done several times (normally four times) per day to test for possible circadian alterations in sleep drive. The individual to be tested usually already has scalp, eye, and sub-mental (under the chin) electrodes applied for overnight sleep recording. They then lie down on a comfortable bed in a darkened and temperature-controlled room and are asked to try to sleep. EEG is monitored continuously for 20 min so that when they fall asleep we can determine what stage of sleep they go into (see Figure 2.6). This can be especially helpful for the diagnosis of narcolepsy, for these patients often enter REM sleep soon after falling asleep.

The MSLT can also be used to detect the sedative effects of drugs such as antidepressants and the carry-over effects of hypnotics with a long half-life, both of which shorten the time to sleep. It is being used more and more as a test for new agents that promote wakefulness (see Chapter 9).

A variant of this test is the Maintenance of Wakefulness Test, in which the subject is prepared in the same way and put into the same room, but is now asked to stay awake for as long as possible. This test may be more sensitive to individuals who have a great propensity to sleep—normal people when instructed to stay awake can usually do so.

Guidelines on exercise and caffeine consumption, etc. between tests are laid down so that they yield interpretable results. If subjects fall asleep during either of these tests, they are usually woken after 1–2 min to reduce the loss of the S function

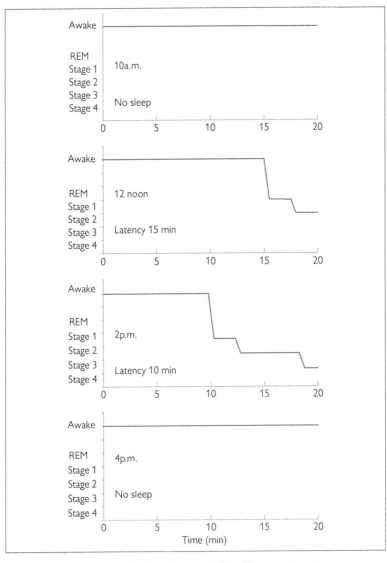

Figure 2.6 Multiple Sleep Latency Test (MSLT) in a normal subject. These are miniature hypnograms showing waking and sleeping over four 20-min sleep opportunities during the day. The sleep propensity is increased after lunch, and the average sleep latency for the day and the previous night (when the subject went to sleep after 10 min) is 15 min, which is normal.

(see Chapter 1), which would make the next test less informative. However, if there is any question of narcolepsy, the MSLT must be continued for the full 20 min to check whether there are REM periods near sleep onset (see Chapter 5).

2.6.4 Overnight video recording

This can usually be done so that PSG and video images can be synchronized, and it is most useful in the differential diagnosis of parasomnias.

2.7 When would these investigations be done?

This varies between sleep centres. In the USA, PSG is widely used, but in the UK and other European countries, home recordings are more commonly used. In each chapter about particular sleep disorders, the usefulness of investigations is described.

References

Buysse DJ, Reynolds CF III, Monk TH, Berman SR, Kupfer DJ (1989). The Pittsburgh Sleep Quality Index: a new instrument for psychiatric practice and research. *Psychiatry Res* **28**: 193–213.

Ellis BW, Johns MW, Lancaster R, Raptopoulos P, Angelopoulos N, Priest RG (1981). The St. Mary's Hospital sleep questionnaire: a study of reliability. *Sleep* **4**: 93–7.

Johns MW (1991). A new method for measuring daytime sleepiness: the Epworth sleepiness scale. *Sleep* **14**: 540–45.

Parrott AC, Hindmarch I (1978). Factor analysis of a sleep evaluation questionnaire. *Psychol Med* **8**: 325–9.

Rechtschaffen A, Kales A (1968). *A Manual of Standardized Terminology, Techniques and Scoring System for Sleep Stages of Human Subjects*. US Department of Health, Education, and Welfare, Washington, DC.

Smith A, Rich N, Wilson S, Nutt D (2001). *Subjective and Objective Assessment of the Effects of Noise, Noise Sensitivity and Noise Disturbed Sleep on Health*. <http://ince.publisher.ingentaconnect.com/content/ince/incecp/2001/00002001/00000005/art00049>

Chapter 3

Insomnia

Key points

- Insomnia is a major health problem and is associated with low quality of life, a high level of absenteeism from work, and physical and mental illness
- Patients report that sleep is too short, too interrupted, or of poor quality, or a combination of these
- It is important to exclude other sleep disorders as a cause of insomnia: referral to a specialist sleep centre for further assessment may be necessary in cases in which the presentation is unusual or the diagnosis is in doubt
- Overall management approaches aim to acknowledge distress, treat the primary cause, educate the patient about trigger factors, and establish good sleep habits
- Current drug treatments for insomnia are hypnotic agents that affect the gamma-aminobutyric acid (GABA)-A-benzodiazepine receptor
- Several new compounds are currently in development

Insomnia is a major public health problem, as it is a common complaint with major consequences for life satisfaction and work productivity as well as for health. Insomnia is a cause of low quality of life (Leger and Poursain 2005; Chevalier et al 1999), results in a high level of absenteeism from work (Leger et al 2006), and is associated with physical illness, perhaps due to reduced natural immunity (Irwin et al 2003; Burgos et al 2006), as well as with mental illness (see Chapter 7).

It causes much distress to sufferers and is one of the most common reasons why people visit their GPs, which in turn causes concerns for these doctors, who often struggle with its treatment. Insomnia poses two main problems for doctors. First, drug treatments are subject to recommendations and restrictions on length of prescribing, which conflict with the long-term nature of many people's insomnia. Secondly, there is a very limited availability of alternative forms of treatment, such as insomnia-focused psychotherapies.

3.1 What are the symptoms of insomnia?

The complaint of poor sleep includes the following:

- too little sleep
- taking too long to go to sleep

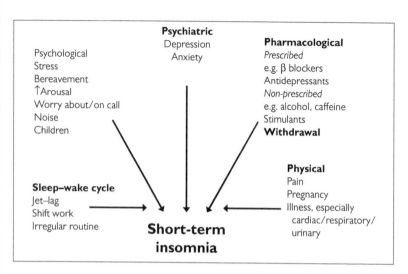

Psychiatric
Depression
Anxiety

Pharmacological
Prescribed
e.g. β blockers
Antidepressants
Non-prescribed
e.g. alcohol, caffeine
Stimulants
Withdrawal

Psychological
Stress
Bereavement
↑Arousal
Worry about/on call
Noise
Children

Physical
Pain
Pregnancy
Illness, especially
    cardiac/respiratory/
    urinary

Sleep–wake cycle
Jet–lag
Shift work
Irregular routine

**Short-term
insomnia**

Figure 3.1 Some precipitating factors in insomnia.

- poor-quality or unrefreshing sleep
- impairment of daytime function—for example, fatigue, poor concentration, memory problems, and low mood

Sleepiness in the daytime (as opposed to fatigue or tiredness) is an *uncommon* feature of insomnia. Usually, when the patient states that they cannot sleep, this means that they have difficulties all the time, not just at night, and if they are sleepy during the day-time, then they may have a circadian rhythm disorder (see Chapter 6).

Sleep onset insomnia is the term used for difficulty in getting to sleep at night, whereas *sleep maintenance insomnia* is the term used for the problem of waking many times dur-ing the night, or waking too early and failing to go back to sleep.

The precipitating factors for insomnia are many and varied (see Figure 3.1). They are usually factors beyond the individual's control that relate either to other problems (e.g. a period of psychological stress, physical or psychiatric illness) or to problems with work or relationships (e.g. irregular sleeping patterns due to shift work). Some precipitating factors are self-inflicted (e.g. choosing activities that lead to irregular sleep, or the use of sleep-disrupting drugs, prescribed or otherwise). Once these temporary factors are no longer present, many people recover their normal sleep patterns, but a proportion go on to develop chronic insomnia.

3.2 How common is insomnia?

Criteria for assessment in population studies vary, but it seems that somewhere around 10–15% of the population have persistent or chronic insomnia (Ohayon *et al* 1997; Roth 2005). The majority of insomniacs are women, with the prevalence increasing with advancing age. Insomnia can be a primary sleep disorder, or secondary to many psychiatric and medical illnesses.

Chapter 3

Insomnia

Insomnia is a major public health problem, as it is a common complaint with major consequences for life satisfaction and work productivity as well as for health. Insomnia is a cause of low quality of life (Leger and Poursain 2005; Chevalier *et al* 1999), results in a high level of absenteeism from work (Leger *et al* 2006), and is associated with physical illness, perhaps due to reduced natural immunity (Irwin *et al* 2003; Burgos *et al* 2006), as well as with mental illness (see Chapter 7).

It causes much distress to sufferers and is one of the most common reasons why people visit their GPs, which in turn causes concerns for these doctors, who often struggle with its treatment. Insomnia poses two main problems for doctors. First, drug treatments are subject to recommendations and restrictions on length of prescribing, which conflict with the long-term nature of many people's insomnia. Secondly, there is a very limited availability of alternative forms of treatment, such as insomnia-focused psychotherapies.

3.1 What are the symptoms of insomnia?

The complaint of poor sleep includes the following:

- too little sleep
- taking too long to go to sleep

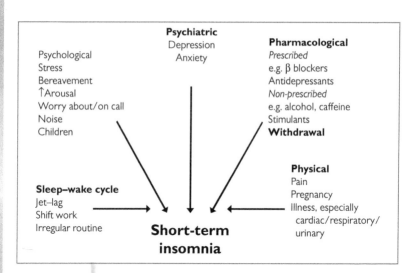

Figure 3.1 Some precipitating factors in insomnia.

- poor-quality or unrefreshing sleep
- impairment of daytime function—for example, fatigue, poor concentration, memory problems, and low mood

Sleepiness in the daytime (as opposed to fatigue or tiredness) is an *uncommon* feature of insomnia. Usually, when the patient states that they cannot sleep, this means that they have difficulties all the time, not just at night, and if they are sleepy during the daytime, then they may have a circadian rhythm disorder (see Chapter 6).

Sleep onset insomnia is the term used for difficulty in getting to sleep at night, whereas *sleep maintenance insomnia* is the term used for the problem of waking many times during the night, or waking too early and failing to go back to sleep.

The precipitating factors for insomnia are many and varied (see Figure 3.1). They are usually factors beyond the individual's control that relate either to other problems (e.g. a period of psychological stress, physical or psychiatric illness) or to problems with work or relationships (e.g. irregular sleeping patterns due to shift work). Some precipitating factors are self-inflicted (e.g. choosing activities that lead to irregular sleep, or the use of sleep-disrupting drugs, prescribed or otherwise). Once these temporary factors are no longer present, many people recover their normal sleep patterns, but a proportion go on to develop chronic insomnia.

3.2 How common is insomnia?

Criteria for assessment in population studies vary, but it seems that somewhere around 10–15% of the population have persistent or chronic insomnia (Ohayon *et al* 1997; Roth 2005). The majority of insomniacs are women, with the prevalence increasing with advancing age. Insomnia can be a primary sleep disorder, or secondary to many psychiatric and medical illnesses.

3.3 What causes insomnia?

Insomnia can be viewed either as a failure of sleep-promoting mechanisms, or as the consequence of these mechanisms being overridden by excess activity of arousal systems. Excessive arousal is a likely explanation when insomnia is associated with anxiety (e.g. before exams) and in patients with anxiety disorders. Indeed, some sleep researchers suggest that primary insomnia may be a form of anxiety disorder in which worry is focused on the need for sleep and the perceived bad consequences of not getting enough sleep, rather than on the more typical topics of finances, children, etc. This worry about sleep leads to arousal, ruminations, and muscle tension that then worsen sleep through a self-fulfilling vicious cycle. Inappropriate and excessive arousal is also a predisposing factor in the insomnia of depression and mania. In dementia and some other neurological disorders, the fragmentation of sleep that leads to insomnia is likely to be due to damage to the sleep-regulating areas of the brain, such as the suprachiasmatic nucleus of the hypothalamus (see Chapter 6).

Common perpetuating factors for insomnia include the following:

- poor sleep habits having been established and allowed to continue
- excessive worrying about sleep
- spending much time and effort 'trying' to sleep.

The last two factors cause more arousal and less likelihood of sleeping; trying to sleep is like trying to forget something, and inevitably leads to a paradoxical worsening of insomnia.

3.4 How is insomnia diagnosed and treated?

Most patients with insomnia present to primary care physicians, and the diagnosis is based on the self-reported subjective symptoms. It is important to exclude other sleep disorders, particularly circadian rhythm disorders, as a cause of insomnia, and therefore a sleep diary will be necessary. Other sleep disorders that need to be excluded are restless legs syndrome (RLS) and parasomnias such as night terrors and sleepwalking. Obstructive sleep apnoea does not usually cause insomnia, but should be seriously considered as a cause of daytime symptoms of 'tiredness' that can mean sleepiness in some patients. (Some suggested questions to help with differential diagnosis can be found in Chapter 2.)

Referral to a specialist sleep centre for further assessment may be necessary in cases where the presentation is unusual or the diagnosis is in doubt, and in that case either actigraphy or polysomnography may be used to assist in the diagnosis.

It is important to treat insomnia, as the condition causes decreased quality of life, is associated with impaired functioning in many areas, and leads to an increased risk of depression, anxiety, and possibly cardiovascular disorders.

The goal of treatment is to lessen suffering and improve daytime function, and the type of treatment should be patient-guided and based on evidence of efficacy. Recommendations for treatment of insomnia (and parasomnias and circadian rhythm disorders) are given in the British Association for Psychopharmacology (BAP) consensus guidelines (Wilson et al 2010).

The initial approach should include the following:

- Acknowledge the patient's distress.
- Treat any precipitating or primary cause if possible.
- Educate the patient about trigger factors for sleep, and reassure them that their sleep will improve.
- Establish good sleep habits.

However, chronic long-term insomnia may not respond to this approach. Care should be taken to identify and treat depressive and anxiety disorders in this group of patients. A treatment algorithm from the BAP consensus guidelines on insomnia treatment is shown in Figure 3.2.

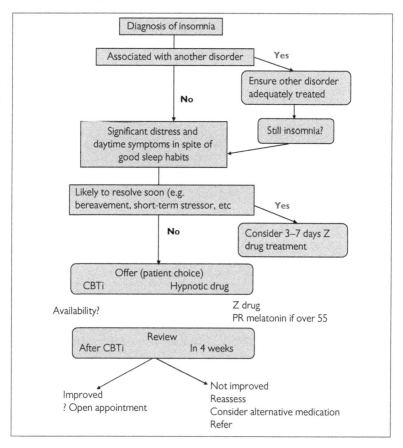

Figure 3.2 Treatment algorithm from the British Association for Psychopharmacology consensus guidelines for treatment of insomnia.

In the treatment of long-term insomnia, the most important factor to be addressed is anxiety about the experience and consequences of (poor) sleep. This often arises from conditioned behaviours that predispose to heightened arousal and tension at bedtime. In insomnia, a cycle has often been established in which insomnia itself leads to the bedroom becoming associated (by conditioning) with not sleeping, thereby perpetuating the problem. As insomnia develops, automatic negative thoughts about the sleeping process begin to occur in the evening. Cognitive behavioural therapy is helpful for dealing with these thoughts and attitudes, and this psychological intervention treatment together with education and sleep hygiene measures as described earlier is the treatment of choice for long-term primary insomnia (Espie 1999). However, the availability of these therapies is often limited, and some patients are unwilling or unable to engage with them.

In some patients with insomnia, the perception of poor sleep is borne out completely by objective evidence—for example, information from a relative or subsequently evidence from actigraphy or polysomnography. However, in most patients there is a degree of underestimation of how much time they were actually asleep, because lying awake with little sensory input makes time go very slowly. A few patients report that they get no sleep at all, or perhaps only a few minutes of sleep, yet the evidence from carers or from polysomnography is that they actually sleep relatively normally. This phenomenon is called sleep misperception, and it can be quite difficult to get the individual concerned to understand the mismatch between their subjective experiences and the physiological measures. In these cases, it is usually best to attempt appropriate psychological therapies, which also include elements aimed at coping in the daytime.

3.5 **Psychological approaches**

Successful psychological treatment involves a combination of information about sleep and good sleep habits, behavioural techniques, and cognitive therapy, focusing on negative automatic thoughts about sleeping (Espie *et al* 2007; Morin and Espie 2003).

3.5.1 **Good sleep habits**

This advice, although seemingly just common sense, is in fact aimed at strengthening the circadian (body clock) and homeostatic (recovery) drives to sleep and minimizing the arousal interferences described in Chapter 1.

- Keep regular bedtimes and rising times.
  This helps both processes, by resynchronizing the clock each day and by ensuring that the time since the last sleep has been long enough to maximize the recovery process.
- Take daytime (but not evening) exercise.
  Physical activity helps to synchronize the clock, but may increase arousal if takes place in the evening.
- Ensure morning exposure to daylight.
  Daylight in the morning is the most powerful synchronizer of the clock.

- Reduce or stop daytime napping.
  This prevents sapping of the recovery drive.
- Avoid stimulants, alcohol, and cigarettes in the late afternoon and evening.
  These all have effects on arousal processes.
- Establish a bedtime routine—'wind down.'
  This minimizes arousal at bedtime.

3.5.2 Behavioural techniques

3.5.2.1 *Stimulus control*

This seeks to minimize environmental cues that may inhibit sleep or strengthen associations in the mind between being in bed and being awake. These include the following:

- continually watching the clock during the night
- using the bed/bedroom for activities other than sleeping—for example, reading, watching TV, or using a mobile phone for texting or surfing the Internet
- staying in bed when awake.

3.5.2.2 *Sleep restriction*

This technique aims to increase sleep efficiency (time asleep as a percentage of time in bed) (see Figure 3.3) Patients are encouraged to assess how much time on average they have actually slept, say during the past week, and then aim to restrict their time in bed to that period. Therefore if they get only 5 h of sleep a night, they choose a preferred getting-up time and must then not try to sleep until 5 h before that time (their new bedtime). They need to use an effective alarm clock for the preferred waking time and reinforce this with help from family members, etc., if necessary. Thus sleep efficiency is increased and eventually the time in bed may be increased gradually. This takes a lot of planning; usually less than 5 h in bed is not recommended, and the technique can cause increased daytime problems for a while, so needs to be carefully supervised by a trained health professional.

3.5.2.3 *Relaxation training*

This is aimed at first learning imagery and muscle relaxation techniques in the daytime, and then developing skills to trigger the relaxed feeling without the therapist or the tape/CD, so that they can be used when sleep is desired.

3.5.3 Cognitive techniques

3.5.3.1 *Cognitive behavioural therapy (CBT)*

This is carried out by trained therapists and aims to change thinking so that not sleeping does not give rise to arousing negative thoughts. These thoughts are common in patients with insomnia—for instance, thinking that they will fail to perform well at work the next day because they are not asleep now.

3.5.3.2 *Rehearsal and planning session*

Patients are encouraged to set aside a short period (about 15 min) in the early evening, after their evening meal, in which they can review the day's activities, write down

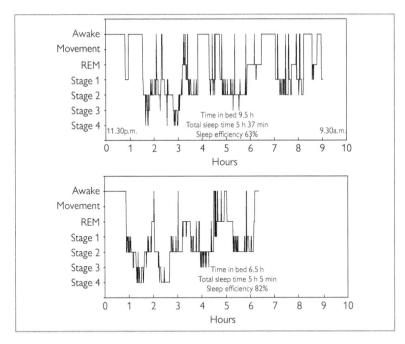

Figure 3.3 Bedtime restriction improves sleep efficiency. In the upper hypnogram, the patient spent 9.5 h in bed, slept for about 5.5 h, and had a sleep efficiency of 63%. Restricting time in bed to 6.5 h reduced sleep to just over 5 h but increased sleep efficiency to 82%, and the patient reported an improvement in sleep quality.

their achievements and plans, and write down positive steps to be taken the next day to resolve problems. No actual work should be done, just planning—for instance, whether to allow a teenager to go out at the weekend (e.g. resolve to discuss this with someone else tomorrow afternoon and make the decision then), or failure to write to the bank today (e.g. resolve to deal with this at 8.30 a.m. tomorrow).

3.5.3.3 *Paradoxical intent*

This is sometimes offered as a strategy that patients can try—it means trying to remain awake in a comfortable bed in the dark. Concentrating on this can sometimes allow sleep to occur.

3.6 Drugs for insomnia

3.6.1 Drugs that act at the GABA-A benzodiazepine receptor

Most of the drugs that are used in insomnia act as agonists at the GABA-A-benzodiazepine receptor and have side effects that include muscle relaxation, memory impairment, and ataxia. This may not be a problem when the patient is asleep, but if it is necessary to get up during the night or if the action of the drug is prolonged past the getting-up time, these effects become very important. Those with a longer duration of action are likely to affect memory, concentration, and performance in skills such as driving, and they will also have enduring anxiolytic and muscle-relaxing effects.

Z-drugs and short-acting benzodiazepines are efficacious for insomnia, and adverse events and carry-over effects are fewer and less serious with decreasing half-lives, so care should be taken to choose a drug with the right timing of onset of action and elimination (see Chapter 9). Care should be taken when prescribing them for patients with comorbid sleep-related breathing disorders such as obstructive sleep apnoea syndrome (see Section 3.6.2), which is exacerbated by benzodiazepines. A very important point is that alcohol potentiates the effects of these drugs, and patients should be made aware that if they have had a drink in the evening, their sleeping pill will have greater and longer-lasting effects, which may have an impact on their driving the next day.

Zopiclone has a half-life of 6–8 h and is an effective drug for both initial and maintenance insomnia. Zolpidem and zaleplon have a fast onset (30–60 min) and a short duration of action, with half-lives of 3 h for zolpidem and 2 h for zaleplon, so are useful for onset insomnia. Studies in volunteers have shown that zaleplon has no effect on psychomotor skills, including driving skills, when taken at least 5 h before testing. This means that it can be taken during the night, either when the patient has been trying to get to sleep for a long time, or if they wake during the night and cannot get back to sleep, without a hangover effect. It is the only prescribable hypnotic that can be used in this way. Patients find it reassuring, because it means that they are not committed to taking a drug every night, but they feel that they have a remedy available 'in case', which increases their confidence about sleeping and reduces their anxiety. The shortest-acting benzodiazepines are temazepam, loprazolam, and lormetazepam, with half-lives of up to 12 h.

Topics that worry patients and their doctors when considering sleeping tablets are those of tolerance, dependence, and withdrawal. These topics are explained more fully in Chapter 9. We have found that chronic insomnia patients can be frightened by their experience of stopping sleeping pills, when there is almost always a short-term rebound of poor sleep, and they interpret this as a pressing need to resume taking them. When it is explained that this rebound is likely to occur even in good sleepers in research studies, they often respond positively. For patients who wish to stop their hypnotics, various strategies are available. One is to encourage intermittent use of short-acting hypnotics, so that the patient knows that they will get a good night's sleep two or three times a week with medication. Another strategy is to encourage dose tapering over a short period, with education of the patient about rebound insomnia. Planning this taper is important, and many patients prefer to use a period of leave from work, or recruit help with family responsibilities for the period when they expect their sleep to be temporarily worse. Treatments that have been shown to improve symptoms in chronic insomnia are those involving psychological intervention, such as cognitive behavioural therapy (CBT) (see Section 3.5.3), and if patients are taught some of these techniques, they may find reduction of the hypnotic medication easier.

Despite these efforts, there will be some patients who continue to complain that their insomnia responds only to drugs. In such cases, the patient and clinician together need to weigh up the risks and benefits of remaining on medication, bearing in mind

the possible risk of the patient using alcohol (or unprescribed drugs) as an alternative. An antidepressant drug may be tried (see Section 3.6.2); the patient should be stabilized on a standard antidepressant dose before withdrawal of the hypnotic is started.

3.6.2 Other drugs used in insomnia

The quest for new drug treatments in insomnia is being pursued with some vigour, and there are several new compounds that show promise (see Chapter 9) but have yet to be compared with currently available treatments. The findings of a study with the active (S) enantiomer of zopiclone (eszopiclone, licensed in the USA) are interesting; in a placebo-controlled trial, efficacy was maintained over 6 months (Krystal et al 2003), and there are now efficacy data for up to 12 months (Roth et al 2005). This is the first time that long-term controlled data has been available showing continued efficacy of a hypnotic, which will be reassuring to patients and their treating doctors.

There is no objective evidence that very low doses of tricyclic antidepressants such as amitriptyline improve sleep in primary insomnia. One reason for not using them is that these drugs are the commonest cause of suicide by self-poisoning with drugs (Nutt 2005). In depression, mirtazapine is useful in patients with marked insomnia as a symptom. In insomniac patients who are not depressed, antidepressant drugs with 5-HT2-blocking effects may occasionally be effective. There have also been reports of selective serotonin reuptake inhibitors (SSRIs) ameliorating long-term insomnia, presumably because their anxiolytic or anti-obsessional effects help to stop the evening anxiety and ruminations about sleep.

The exogenous administration of melatonin, the hormone produced by the pineal gland during darkness, has been investigated for the treatment of insomnia, but the results appear to be inconclusive (Buscemi et al 2005), although melatonin is useful in circadian rhythm disorders. Its half-life is short, and a slow-release formulation of melatonin has been licensed on the basis of improved sleep continuity and daytime well-being in people aged over 55 years with insomnia (Lemoine et al, 2007; Wade et al, 2007). It is thought that this age group may benefit because the endogenous melatonin secretion rhythm is reduced. Melatonin produces shortening of sleep latency, and shows no cognitive, motor, or respiratory impairing effects.

Most proprietary (over-the-counter, OTC) sleep remedies contain antihistamines. The only antihistamine with efficacy in a controlled trial is promethazine (available OTC as Sominex®), which reduces sleep onset latency and awakenings during the night after a single dose, but there have been no studies lasting longer than one night. Most antihistamine sedatives have a relatively long action and may cause daytime sedation.

There have been very few randomized clinical trials of herbal sleep aids (see Gyllenhaal et al 2000), and so far the evidence for their efficacy is inconsistent.

References

Burgos I, Richter L, Klein T et al (2006). Increased nocturnal interleukin-6 excretion in patients with primary insomnia: a pilot study. Brain Behav Immun **20**: 246–53.

Buscemi N, Vandermeer B, Hooton N et al (2005). The efficacy and safety of exogenous melatonin for primary sleep disorders. A meta-analysis. *J Gen Intern Med* **20**: 1151–8.

Chevalier H, Los F, Boichut D et al (1999). Evaluation of severe insomnia in the general population: results of a European multinational survey. *J Psychopharmacol* **13**: S21–4.

Espie CA (1999). Cognitive behaviour therapy as the treatment of choice for primary insomnia. *Sleep Med Rev* **3**: 97–9.

Espie CA, MacMahon KM, Kelly HL et al (2007). Randomized clinical effectiveness trial of nurse-administered small-group cognitive behavior therapy for persistent insomnia in general practice. *Sleep* **30**: 574–84.

Gyllenhaal C, Merritt SL, Peterson SD, Block KI, Gochenour T (2000). Efficacy and safety of herbal stimulants and sedatives in sleep disorders. *Sleep Med Rev* **4**: 229–51.

Irwin M, Clark C, Kennedy B, Christian GJ, Ziegler M (2003). Nocturnal catecholamines and immune function in insomniacs, depressed patients, and control subjects. *Brain Behav Immun* **17**: 365–72.

Krystal AD, Walsh JK, Laska E et al (2003). Sustained efficacy of eszopiclone over 6 months of nightly treatment: results of a randomized, double-blind, placebo-controlled study in adults with chronic insomnia. *Sleep* **26**: 793–9.

Leger D, Poursain B (2005). An international survey of insomnia: under-recognition and under-treatment of a polysymptomatic condition. *Curr Med Res Opin* **21**: 1785–92.

Leger D, Massuel MA, Metlaine A (2006). Professional correlates of insomnia. *Sleep* **29**: 171–8.

Lemoine P, Nir T, Laudon M, Zisapel N (2007). Prolonged-release melatonin improves sleep quality and morning alertness in insomnia patients aged 55 years and older and has no withdrawal effects. *J Sleep Res* **16**: 372–80.

Morin CM, Espie CA (2003). *Insomnia: a Clinician's Guide to Assessment and Treatment.* Kluwer, New York.

Nutt DJ (2005). Death by tricyclic: the real antidepressant scandal? *J Psychopharmacol* **19**: 123–4.

Ohayon MM, Caulet M, Priest RG, Guilleminault C (1997). DSM-IV and ICSD-90 insomnia symptoms and sleep dissatisfaction. *Br J Psychiatry* **171**: 382–388.

Roth T (2005). Prevalence, associated risks, and treatment patterns of insomnia. *J Clin Psychiatry* **66 (Suppl. 9)**: 10–13.

Roth T, Walsh JK, Krystal A, Wessel T, Roehrs TA (2005). An evaluation of the efficacy and safety of eszopiclone over 12 months in patients with chronic primary insomnia. *Sleep Med* **6**: 487–95.

Wade AG, Ford I, Crawford G et al (2007). Efficacy of prolonged release melatonin in insomnia patients aged 55–80 years: quality of sleep and next-day alertness outcomes. *Curr Med Res Opin* **23**: 2597–605.

Wilson SJ, Nutt DJ, Alford C et al (2010). British Association for Psychopharmacology consensus statement on evidence-based treatment of insomnia, parasomnias and circadian rhythm disorders. *J Psychopharmacol* **24**: 1577–601.

Hypersomnia

- Excessive daytime sleepiness or *hypersomnia* can be caused by a number of factors, including insufficient sleep syndrome, depression, neurological disorders, and drug side effects
- Hypersomnia can also be caused by a primary sleep disorder such as obstructive sleep apnoea, narcolepsy, idiopathic or recurrent hypersomnia, or circadian rhythm disorder

Hypersomnia is the term used for feeling sleepy during the day. The distinction between fatigue (feelings of tiredness, lethargy, and lack of energy or drive) and sleepiness (the tendency to fall asleep) is important, and there are questionnaires that help with this distinction. Hypersomnia or excessive daytime sleepiness is prevalent in the general population, with a sizable proportion of adults (37%) reporting that they are so sleepy during the day that this interferes with their daily activities on a few days a month or more, and 16% reporting that it impairs their activities on a few days per week or more (National Sleep Foundation 2002). This figure rises in adolescents and young adults, perhaps due to their lifestyles.

Lack of sleep without any underlying disease (insufficient sleep syndrome) is probably the most frequent cause of daytime sleepiness, with depression, neurological disorders, and drug effects being the next most frequent causes. When it occurs as a symptom of a primary sleep disorder, sleepiness may be related to:

- fragmentation of nocturnal sleep (e.g. by breathing-related disorders, movement disorders, or parasomnias)
- intrusion of sleep phenomena into the awake state (e.g. in narcolepsy)
- disturbances of circadian rhythms (e.g. in delayed sleep phase syndrome).

It is important that health professionals are familiar with the characteristics and causes of these.

4.1 Obstructive sleep apnoea syndrome (OSAS)

This is the most common breathing disorder that gives rise to daytime sleepiness. In this disorder, collapse of the upper airway during sleep leads to a state of hypoxia and hypercapnia (elevated carbon dioxide levels) that activates the brainstem, leading to an arousal that increases breathing and rectifies the problem. These patients are often large men with fat necks who snore loudly. The arousals are often associated with sharp intake of deep breaths and splutterings that cause the partner a great deal of concern and auditory discomfort, and often lead to their having poor sleep, too. In severe cases, people in adjacent rooms can be disturbed by the loud noises during the OSAS sufferer's sleep.

These hypoxic/hypercapnic arousals can occur up to hundreds of times each night, causing significant sleep deprivation that in turn results in sleepiness during the day. For this reason, OSAS is a major public health problem which has a huge effect on the quality of life of sufferers and their partners, and which increases the risk of road traffic accidents by up to 11-fold (George 2004). OSAS is also an independent risk factor for cardiovascular disease.

4.1.1 What are the symptoms of OSAS?

- The presenting symptom is usually excessive daytime sleepiness.
- Sometimes the bed partner has requested referral because of worry about other symptoms.
- Loud snoring.
- Interruptions in breathing at night.
- Breathing resumed with loud noises such as gasps, mumbling, or violent movements.
- The patient is often unaware of their night-time behaviour.
- OSAS can cause marital problems.
- Sometimes there is dry mouth, sore throat, or headache in the morning.

The severity of subjective sleepiness can be estimated with the Epworth Sleepiness Scale (see Chapter 2).

4.1.2 How common is OSAS?

The risk of OSAS is increased in males with obesity, particularly those with upper-body obesity and a large neck. It is also increased to a lesser extent in people with craniofacial abnormalities, Down's syndrome, large tonsils/adenoids, and in disorders such as chronic obstructive pulmonary disease and stroke.

The prevalence of the disorder depends on the diagnostic criteria used. In individuals with moderate to severe disease who have clear sleepiness, the prevalence is probably about 0.5% in a UK population of middle-aged men with a mean body mass index (BMI) of about 25 kg/m^2, and in a similar population with a mean BMI of 27 kg/m^2 it increases to about 1.5% (Stradling and Crosby 1991). If the criteria are defined using polysomnography as having more than five apnoeas per hour plus daytime sleepiness, then the prevalence rises to about 4% in males and 2% in females in a US population with a mean BMI of about 30 kg/m^2 (Young et al 1993). Recent studies have highlighted the increased obesity among the general population, and therefore the increased risk of OSAS (Usmani et al 2013).

4.1.3 What causes OSAS?

The principal mechanism is a narrowed upper airway due to anatomical factors. When we breathe in, negative pressure in the upper airway tends to make it narrower. To compensate for this, there is a negative pressure reflex via phasic muscles affecting the airway, primarily the genioglossus, which protrudes the tongue. These muscles contract with each inspiration in order to stiffen the airway and make it less likely to decrease in size. There are also muscles that maintain tone throughout the breathing cycle. The activity of both tonic and phasic muscles decreases during sleep, and therefore the airway is more likely to narrow when breathing in. Turbulence in a narrowed pharynx causes snoring.

OSAS sufferers have a narrower airway to start with, so it is more likely to collapse. The diaphragm continues to try to pull air in, but there is no airflow. Blood oxygen levels decrease and carbon dioxide levels increase, and the autonomic reflex via medullary chemoreceptors causes an alarm signal, which leads to awakening. There is a transient increase in blood pressure at the end of each arousal, even in normal arousals in healthy people, but in OSA this is much larger, between 30 and 50 mmHg systolic pressure. The mechanism underlying this increase is not yet known (McArdle *et al* 2007), but is probably related to the hypoxic events and the surges of the autonomic nervous system that occur during the arousals, as well as to the poor quality of the sleep.

Sleep is therefore fragmented, restless, and inadequate, leading to daytime sleepiness and napping, and in some cases falling asleep at the wheel of the car or lorry, with disastrous consequences.

4.1.4 How do we diagnose and treat OSAS?

OSAS is diagnosed and treated by specialist sleep disorder clinics and by respiratory physicians with a special interest in sleep. In some countries, and occasionally in the UK, patients will be admitted to hospital for overnight sleep studies, which include measures of airflow, blood oxygen saturation, and respiratory effort, and less often full polysomnography, including electroencephalogram (EEG) sleep staging. More often these days there will be a limited home sleep study, which records a few physiological variables related to breathing (e.g. airflow, oximetry from the ear lobe or finger), followed by more extensive inpatient studies if the diagnosis is in doubt. Usually an index of breathing pauses per hour, called the Apnoea/Hypopnoea Index (AHI), is derived from these studies.

The treatment that has been shown to be most effective is weight reduction. In fact, in a cohort that was studied twice 4 years apart (Peppard *et al* 2000), a 10% weight gain predicted a 32% increase in overnight apnoeas, and a 10% loss in weight predicted a 26% decrease. However, achieving this weight reduction often proves difficult, and the most widely used treatment is continuous positive airway pressure (CPAP). This involves the patient wearing a nasal mask at night through which a machine blows air at a prescribed pressure titrated to the patient's requirements to keep the pharynx open. This continuous stream of air prevents the airway from collapsing during sleep. CPAP treatment can be highly effective in the treatment of obstructive sleep apnoea, and the severity of symptoms, rather than the objectively measured AHI, seems to be the best predictor of outcome. Improvement in the quality of sleep and quality of life are often noticed after only a few nights' use. Patients are often initially reluctant to use this therapy, because the apparatus looks a little daunting and feels strange. Fitting the mask is important, and some patients try several masks before a suitable fit is found. Some individuals quickly adjust to the treatment, others struggle for longer periods, and some discontinue treatment entirely.

In many patients, the disturbed breathing is improved but there is residual daytime sleepiness. In these individuals, it is worth considering the use of the wakefulness-promoting drug modafinil (see Chapter 9) to increase wakefulness in the daytime. Modafinil has a licence for this purpose in the UK and the USA, and studies have shown improvements in alertness (see Keating and Raffin 2005).

4.2 Narcolepsy

Narcolepsy is a chronic lifelong condition that has severe consequences for education, work, and relationships.

4.2.1 What are the symptoms of narcolepsy?

- Daytime sleepiness, often with sudden onset of sleep—'sleep attacks'
- Cataplexy—sudden loss of skeletal muscle
- Hypnagogic/hypnopompic hallucinations
- Fragmented night-time sleep

Narcolepsy results from a disturbance of the brain mechanisms that control sleep and waking. In particular, there is intrusion of elements of rapid eye movement (REM) sleep into wakefulness.

- Excessive daytime sleepiness is the most common presenting complaint. It occurs alone or in combination with other symptoms, and almost always develops in the course of the disorder. This refers both to a continuous feeling of sleepiness and to the strong, sometimes irresistible desire for sleep, which occurs at intervals through the day. These naps, or 'sleep attacks', last for several minutes but seldom more than an hour, and can happen up to five times a day.
- Cataplexy—this is the loss of skeletal muscle tone and power in response to emotion, especially laughter, amusement, anger, elation, and surprise. The patient is usually fully aware during the attacks, which generally last for less than a minute but sometimes for a few minutes. When this loss of muscle power is total, the patient falls to the ground, but cataplexy is often partial, with, for example, head nodding, sagging of the jaw, and weakening of the knees. Irregular twitching of the face or limbs is sometimes seen with the gradual return of muscle tone. Many affected individuals learn to suppress emotion in order to minimize the risk of an attack.
- Hypnagogic/hypnopompic hallucinations—these are vivid, dream-like experiences that occur at the start or end of sleep, whether in the daytime or at night. Patients estimate that they last up to several minutes, and often say that they have difficulty in deciding what is real and what is dreaming.
- Fragmented night-time sleep is commonly reported, and it seems that if all episodes of sleep over a period of 24 h are summed in these patients, the time spent actually asleep may be similar to that in a normal population.

All parasomnias (see Chapter 5) are increased in narcolepsy, particularly sleep paralysis. Additional symptoms described in this condition are automatic behaviour in performing tasks at times of increased sleepiness, with little or no recall of the episode, sleep drunkenness (a period of confused behaviour on awakening), visual disturbances, and a range of cognitive symptoms from poor concentration and forgetfulness to depressed mood.

Many of the psychosocial consequences of narcolepsy are a result of daytime sleepiness and are in principle amenable to treatment.

4.2.2 How common is narcolepsy?

The prevalence of narcolepsy in European populations has been estimated to be 3–4 in 10,000. Onset can occur at any age, but is most frequent in the second decade of life. The majority of sufferers have a particular tissue type of the human leukocyte antigen (HLA DQB1*0602), but so do 18–35% of the general population. Family members have a very slightly increased risk (by 1–2%), but a clear-cut family history is the exception.

4.2.3 What is the aetiology of narcolepsy?

Great strides have been made in finding out the underlying mechanisms of sleep and wakefulness regulation with the discovery in the last 10 years that peptides in the brain called orexins (also known as hypocretins) have a major role. The neurons that synthesize orexins are present in the hypothalamus, the seat of circadian regulation, and their axons project to many of the key brainstem and midbrain centres that regulate sleep and arousal. Orexin release is associated with being awake and alert and stabilizing the awake state. For many decades we have known that some animal strains also show narcolepsy and cataplexy, especially some dogs. More recently, a mouse mutation of the orexin-1-receptor gene has been found that is associated with a narcoleptic type of picture, because the receptor is insensitive to the natural neurotransmitter orexin. Humans with narcolepsy do not have this receptor mutation, but it has been found that there is a lack of orexin in the cerebrospinal fluid (CSF), and at postmortem there appear to be few or no orexin cells in the hypothalamus. Since the onset of the disease peaks in adolescence and patients have a common HLA type, it is thought that the cause of orexin cell death may be an infection whereby the immune response to the infecting agents cross-reacts with some elements of the orexin neurons, leading to an autoimmune attack on these cells and their destruction. Some other neurological disorders—for example, Sydenham's chorea—are similarly of autoimmune origin, although in this case the damage is to dopaminergic neurons in the basal ganglia.

4.2.4 How do we diagnose narcolepsy?

Narcolepsy is usually treated by specialist sleep centres or by neurologists with a special interest in sleep disorders. The combination of excessive daytime sleepiness and unambiguous cataplexy makes the diagnosis of narcolepsy highly probable. Without cataplexy the diagnosis is less definite, and therefore the investigation that is needed is a Multiple Sleep Latency Test (MSLT; see Chapter 2), which is always preceded by an overnight sleep recording (polysomnography). In narcolepsy, the dysregulation of REM control means that these patients will fall rapidly into REM sleep soon after falling asleep (sleep-onset REM). If the MSLT is short (showing increased sleepiness) and there are sleep-onset REM periods in at least two of the five tests, then a diagnosis of narcolepsy is very likely (see Figure 4.1).

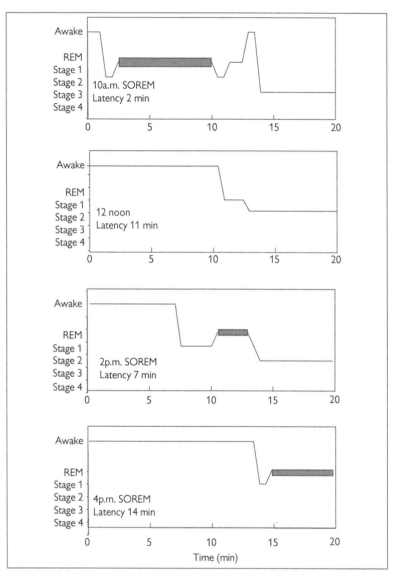

Figure 4.1 Example of a multiple sleep latency test in narcolepsy. These are miniature hypnograms (see Chapter 2 for normal subject). At the 10 a.m., 2 p.m., and 4 p.m. sleep opportunities the subject had a period of REM sleep (thick line) near sleep onset (SOREM). The mean sleep latency is 8 min.

4.2.5 **Treatment**

Because of the lifelong and life-impairing nature of narcolepsy, patients should be given information about narcolepsy at the time of diagnosis, and this information should also be made available to family members, friends, teachers and employers, and healthcare professionals. Patients should be advised to try to get adequate amounts of nocturnal sleep, taken in a regular fashion. Where possible, planned daytime naps are sometimes useful, so people with narcolepsy should be enabled to take naps at school and work if this improves their symptoms or performance. More detailed treatment guidelines are available (Billiard *et al* 2006).

Daytime sleepiness is usually treated with the wakefulness-promoting drug modafinil, or with a stimulant such as dexamfetamine or methylphenidate. These stimulants have an advantage over modafinil in that they also reduce cataplexy, perhaps because they have effects on the 5HT system. However, cataplexy is usually treated separately either with the mixed noradrenaline 5HT uptake blocker venlafaxine or with clomipramine, or selective serotonin reuptake inhibitors (SSRIs) (e.g. fluoxetine). In recent years, a new treatment for cataplexy has been developed, namely sodium oxybate. This works in an entirely different fashion, as it is used at night to treat the disruption of sleep continuity seen in narcolepsy. It is a difficult drug to use, as it has a very short half-life, so the patient needs to wake up during the night to take a second dose. However, it has a profound effect in consolidating REM sleep and increasing slow-wave sleep (SWS), and reduces cataplexy and sometimes daytime sleepiness. More information on these drugs can be found in Chapter 9.

Treatment should be monitored carefully by the specialist, and usually these patients are seen at least every 6 months for life.

4.2.6 **Narcolepsy in children**

Although this book does not cover sleep disorders in children, the peak onset of narcolepsy is in the second decade of life, and knowledge of some of the symptoms encountered in childhood may be useful when taking a history. A more complete description has been given by Stores (2006).

- Symptoms of narcolepsy are seen in childhood or adolescence in at least one-third of cases, and can occur as early as 2 years of age.
- Sleepiness may take the form of over-long night-time sleep or persistence of daytime naps; it may also cause *increased* activity, which does not occur in adults with narcolepsy.
- Cataplexy, especially partial forms, may be misinterpreted as silly/attention-seeking behaviour or clumsiness. Sometimes, frank episodes can be confused with syncope (common in adolescence).
- Children can suffer from the effects of disrupted sleep on learning, mood, behaviour at home or in school, and social and other activities. They can also experience distress, embarrassment, and ridicule because of the symptoms.

Treatments are similar to those used in adults; stimulants have been extensively used in children with attention deficit disorders, so are known to be safe in the younger age group.

4.3 Other causes of daytime sleepiness

4.3.1 Idiopathic hypersomnia

If symptoms of long sleep or excessive daytime sleepiness occur without fulfilling diagnostic criteria for a primary sleep disorder, or do not appear to be psychiatric, neurological, or pharmacological in origin, then they are labelled idiopathic. There is some evidence that this condition runs in families, suggesting genetic factors may play a role.

Treatment to improve symptoms depends on severity and degree of impairment, but if work or study is significantly impaired, then treatment is warranted. The approach is similar to that for treating sleepiness in narcolepsy in that stimulants or modafinil can be used, although probably not sodium oxybate. Improving nocturnal sleep using sleep hygiene measures or an appropriate hypnotic (see Chapter 9) may also be helpful.

4.3.2 Recurrent hypersomnia

Kleine–Levin syndrome (KLS) is a rare disease in which there are recurrent episodes of hypersomnia and sometimes behavioural or cognitive disturbances, compulsive eating behaviour, and sometimes hypersexuality. In between the episodes, the patient is quite normal. The disease predominantly affects adolescent males. Although there is no population-based information about KLS prevalence, it is generally considered to be an exceptionally rare disease. The largest case series is a worldwide database of 186 sufferers, which has provided the best information available to date (Arnulf *et al* 2005).

About 40% of patients report an infection at the start of the disease, but when an infectious agent has been identified (which has been rare), it differed from one patient to another. However, this association with infection does suggest that, like narcolepsy, KLS may have an autoimmune component.

The duration of the disease is about 4–8 years, and a long-term follow-up study reported that 25 patients were in good health several years after the cessation of their KLS episodes (Gadoth *et al* 2001).

Treatments which decrease sleepiness during episodes are drugs such as the amphetamines, but only half of patients show any improvement. Attempts to reduce the frequency or number of episodes have been less successful, with only lithium prophylaxis having any effect, and that only in about 40% of those treated. The risk benefit of this in young adults must obviously be carefully considered, and advice relating to regular sleep habits and avoiding excessive night-time activities such as raves should be given.

4.3.3 Circadian rhythm disorders

Disorders of circadian rhythm occur when the sleep–wake pattern is out of synchrony with either the desired timetable of the patient or normal patterns of society. They cause people to be sleepy at times when they want to be awake. A more detailed description of these disorders is given in Chapter 6.

4.3.4 Restless legs syndrome/periodic limb movement disorder

These movement disorders (see Chapter 8) may cause frequent arousals from sleep if they are severe, and therefore fragment sleep as in OSAS, with consequent daytime sleepiness.

Table 4.1 Severity criteria for daytime sleepiness (American Sleep Disorders Association)

Severity	Examples of situations where it becomes evident	Frequency	Social/occupational impairment	Associated MSLT latency (min)
Mild	Watching television, reading while lying down in a quiet room, or being a passenger in a moving vehicle	Less than daily	Mild	10–15
Moderate	During concerts, film/theatre performances, group meetings, or when driving	Daily	Moderate	5–10
Severe	During eating, direct personal conversation, driving, walking, or physical activities	Daily	Marked	< 5

Box 4.1 Key questions when faced with a patient omplaining of hypersomnia

- Does the patient sleep longer at weekends? (Could indicate insufficient sleep)
- Is the patient male, overweight, and middle-aged? Does he snore loudly? (Could indicate OSAS)
- Does the patient ever go weak at the knees when emotionally aroused—for example, when laughing? (Could indicate cataplexy)

4.4 **Severity of daytime sleepiness**

The American Sleep Disorders Association has recommended some severity criteria for daytime sleepiness (see Table 4.1 and Box 4.1).

References

Arnulf I, Zeitzer JM, File J, Farber N, Mignot E (2005). Kleine–Levin syndrome: a systematic review of 186 cases in the literature. *Brain* **128**: 2763–76.

Billiard M, Bassetti C, Dauvilliers Y et al; EFNS Task Force (2006). EFNS guidelines on management of narcolepsy. *Eur J Neurol* **13**: 1035–48.

Gadoth N, Kesler A, Vainstein G, Peled R, Lavie P (2001). Clinical and polysomnographic characteristics of 34 patients with Kleine–Levin syndrome. *J Sleep Res* **10**: 337–41.

George CF (2004). Sleep. 5: Driving and automobile crashes in patients with obstructive sleep apnoea/hypopnoea syndrome. *Thorax* **59**: 804–7.

Keating GM, Raffin MJ (2005). Modafinil: a review of its use in excessive sleepiness associated with obstructive sleep apnoea/hypopnoea syndrome and shift work sleep disorder. *CNS Drugs* **19**: 785–803.

McArdle N, Hillman D, Beilin L, Watts G (2007). Metabolic risk factors for vascular disease in obstructive sleep apnea: a matched controlled study. *Am J Respir Crit Care Med* **175**: 190–95.

National Sleep Foundation (2002). *2002 'Sleep in America' Poll*. <www.sleepfoundation.org/sites/default/files/2002SleepInAmericaPoll.pdf>

Peppard PE, Young T, Palta M, Dempsey J, Skatrud J (2000). Longitudinal study of moderate weight change and sleep-disordered breathing. *JAMA* **284**: 3015–21.

Stores G (2006). The protean manifestations of childhood narcolepsy and their misinterpretation. *Dev Med Child Neurol* **48**: 307–10.

Stradling JR, Crosby JH (1991). Predictors and prevalence of obstructive sleep apnoea and snoring in 1001 middle-aged men. *Thorax* **46**: 85–90.

Usmani ZA, Chai-Coetzer CL, Antic NA, McEvoy RD (2013). Obstructive sleep apnoea in adults. *Postgrad Med J* **89**: 148–56.

Young T, Palta M, Dempsey J, Skatrud J, Weber S, Badr S (1993). The occurrence of sleep-disordered breathing among middle-aged adults. *N Engl J Med* **328**: 1230–35.

Parasomnias

Parasomnias are unusual episodes or behaviours that occur during sleep and which disturb the patient or others. The classification of these fascinating disorders is easiest to understand by looking at the stage of sleep from which they arise. A clinically relevant feature relates to the ability of the sufferer to remember what has happened; in general, parasomnias arising from deep non-rapid-eye-movement (non-REM) sleep are not remembered clearly by the patient, whereas the ones from REM sleep are. A summary of the features that distinguish the main parasomnias is provided in the following sections. Panic attacks that occur during the night are not uncommon, and are also included, as these may be confused with parasomnias (see Table 5.1).

5.1 Parasomnias that arise from non-REM sleep

5.1.1 Night terrors (also called sleep terrors)

5.1.1.1 *What are the symptoms of night terrors?*

- Recurrent episodes of abrupt awakening, most commonly in the first third of the night, usually with a scream
- Intense fear and signs of autonomic arousal
- Unresponsiveness to comforting
- No detailed recall

Table 5.1 The parasomnias

Parasomnia	Sleep stage	Behaviour	Responsive/ oriented	Recall
Sleepwalking	SWS	Automatic behaviour (e.g. walking around house, to toilet, to get drink, etc.)	No	None
Night terrors	SWS	Screaming, fearful, agitated demeanour, and flight/fight behaviour	No	None, occasionally recollection of fear
Nightmares	REM	During:none After waking: fearful, agitated demeanour	Yes	Recall of frightening dream, knows it was a dream
REM behaviour disorder	REM	During: violent complex actions with vocalization After waking: fearful, agitated demeanour	Unresponsive but quickly awakened Yes	Recall of clear structured dream, usually active, violent, and unpleasant
Panic attack	Transition from wake to sleep or light to deep sleep	Fearful, agitated demeanour	Yes	Full, as daytime panic attack

- On waking from a terror (not common), confusion and disorientation, vague memory of imagery, usually about choking, being trapped, or non-specific fears
- Cause significant distress

Night terrors usually start with a scream or shout. The sufferer sits up in bed and sometimes engages in automatic behaviour associated with fear and escape, such as running out of the room, jumping out of a window, and sometimes running into the street, or with fighting, in which self, companions, or objects can be attacked. In a child, these behaviours can generally be contained, but in an adult they can be dangerous to the sufferer and the sleeping partner. There are many reports in the literature of severe injury (and sometimes death) occurring during the period of confusion following the rise from bed. In addition to the dangerous consequences of automatic behaviour, individuals who have more frequent attacks suffer from serious disruption of sleep. This can markedly impair subsequent daytime functioning, and may lead to significant secondary psychiatric comorbidity, particularly depression and anxiety. Night terrors can therefore cause profound disability.

5.1.1.2 How common are night terrors?

Night terrors are common in children, among whom around 30–40% have at least one episode. The peak age for these is at about 2–3 years, with a gradual diminution up to early adolescence. In some cases, night terrors persist into adult life, but more commonly they recur in the twenties or thirties, often when the subject is experiencing a stressful life period. The prevalence in adults is unknown, as there do not appear to have been any systematic epidemiological studies, and patients usually only present if there has been an adverse event. However, a likely estimate of the prevalence is probably about 2%, and almost all patients have experienced night terrors or sleepwalking as a child. There is no gender difference in prevalence. Up to 80% of sufferers report a family history of either night terrors or sleepwalking. Patients with night terrors have an increased incidence of comorbid psychiatric disorder, particularly anxiety disorders, and in otherwise healthy people they seem to be clustered in periods of increased stress, such as moving away from the family home, starting a new relationship, etc., and are a particular problem when in a new environment such as a hotel room, starting in student accommodation, etc. The occurrence of night terrors and sleepwalking in the same patient is fairly common.

5.1.1.3 *What is the cause?*

The best explanation for the mechanism underlying these terrors is that they are incomplete arousals from slow-wave sleep (SWS), during which cognitive function is 'switched off', allowing the manifestation of behaviour that is driven from subcortical arousal and anxiety centres. However, we do not know what causes the arousals. There is manifestly a constitutional predisposition that suggests a genetic influence, which may make people more susceptible to environmental influences. Pockets of high prevalence of night terrors and sleepwalking have been found—for example, among the settlers of Welsh extraction in Patagonia—which again suggests some genetic basis. Patients with night terrors may have an inability to sustain SWS, which then allows frightening arousals to emerge from the brainstem or limbic areas. In fact, in severe cases where the terrors are frequent and occur every night, patients can be deprived of SWS, because each time they enter SWS it is immediately terminated by a terror (see Figure 5.1). They often report fear at bedtime and rumination about the consequences of an episode during sleep, which gives rise to further anxiety and may predispose to more episodes.

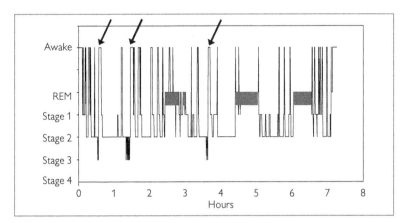

Figure 5.1 Hypnogram of a patient with night terrors. The patient had three episodes during the night (marked with arrows). Each time she entered a period of SWS, she had a terror, thus ending the period, and therefore she was deprived of SWS.

5.1.1.4 *How are night terrors diagnosed and treated?*

The diagnosis is usually made on clinical grounds by a sleep specialist, but in order to be sure of the diagnosis, it is desirable to record an episode during polysomnography with video recording. This can be done in a sleep laboratory or in the person's own home. In both cases, video recording with an infrared camera is used. The terrors usually occur soon after entry into an episode of SWS, and so they commonly happen in the first few hours of sleep when SWS is at its maximum. This helps to differentiate them from nightmares, which usually occur in REM, so they are maximal later in the night.

Having a diagnosis is reassuring to patients, as they often tell us that their families make them feel that they could somehow stop the episodes if they had sufficient self-control! They also report guilt about the effect that the night-time disturbance has on the family, and fear that they will harm themselves or someone else.

Trigger factors should be minimized.

- Alcohol may increase the risk of night terror, because it deepens SWS, especially at the beginning of the night.
- Episodes are more dangerous when the person is sleeping in a strange environment.

For instance, escape behaviour is dependent on the door being in its familiar position in the bedroom, and if it is not, an attempted exit via stairs or a window may cause injury. This explains well-documented cases of people falling out of hotel windows. Many people prepare themselves for this possibility by taking locks with them to secure doors and windows when they are sleeping away from home. Patients who prefer not to take medication every day may wish to use it on an as-needed [pro re nata (prn)] basis at times of high risk like this.

The medication for which there is most evidence is nightly clonazepam (Schenck and Mahowald 1996), a benzodiazepine with a long duration of action, which works by decreasing arousal from sleep (see Chapter 9). Unfortunately, it may also cause daytime hangover effects, and the risk–benefit balance must be clearly discussed. Paroxetine, an antidepressant that increases serotonin function, is also effective (Wilson et al 1997). It can work even after the first dose, which means that the mechanism cannot be the same as that for lifting mood, which usually takes 3–4 weeks. The most likely explanation is a direct pharmacological action to increase serotonin in brainstem regions suppressing ascending arousal pathways. Some patients with severe or nightly terrors will be happy to take this medication on a long-term basis. Others may wish to try it for a few months and see whether the terror 'habit' can be broken. Medication should be tailed off gradually, because there is a risk of rebound after long-term dosing.

5.1.2 **Sleepwalking**

5.1.2.1 *Symptoms of sleepwalking*

- Automatic behaviour at night with the sufferer unresponsive to surroundings and other people
- Most commonly walking around
- Can include other behaviours which are highly familiar to the subject, such as dressing, washing, making tea, arranging possessions

In some cases, the attacks seem to be precipitated by the need to urinate, and the sufferer may leave the bedroom to go the toilet, pass urine while still asleep, and then return to bed without any recollection of this behaviour the next day.

5.1.2.2 *How common is sleepwalking?*

The incidence of sleepwalking is unknown, but it probably has a lifetime prevalence of 15–20%. Patients rarely present for treatment unless there has been injury to self or others. In rare cases, near-death experiences have been reported; for example, one sufferer found himself asleep on a ledge in the middle of a high cliff with no recollection of how he had got there, and he had to be rescued by helicopter. Sleepwalking has a similar clinical course to night terrors, and almost certainly these are both variants of the same underlying pathology.

5.1.2.3 *How is sleepwalking treated?*

Again minimization of trigger factors is important, and making the patient's environment safe is even more crucial for sleepwalkers. As in night terrors, there seems to be no awareness of the outside world, and familiar actions and routes are dangerous when performed or followed in a strange environment. For instance, the sleepwalker's family may want to lock the hotel-room door when on holiday.

Drug treatment is the same as for night terrors, although it is less often required.

5.1.3 **Confusional arousals**

Other behaviours that arise from deep sleep and which show a similar unresponsiveness to external cues are called confusional arousals. They may be accompanied by semi-purposeful movements such as searching for or handling objects in the bedroom. Some people who experience these arousals prepare and eat food during these periods, and because of their unawareness they often eat inappropriate things which are in a usual food-containing place, such as butter or raw meat. This can also be dangerous (e.g. eating the contents of an ashtray). This form of parasomnia has been called sleep eating disorder.

There have been a few reports of sex with the bed partner occurring in an otherwise unresponsive person in the middle of the night. These episodes always occur without the subject getting out of bed, and there is always a history of other confusional arousals. It seems likely that these episodes are part of the spectrum of night terrors and sleepwalking, and they are treated in the same way if they are sufficiently impairing to require interventions.

5.1.4 **Sleep bruxism**

This is also known as *teeth grinding*, and it usually presents to dental practitioners as an erosion of the tooth surface or morning jaw pain or headaches. It does not seem to disrupt sleep subjectively, but the noises made can be quite loud and often annoy the bed partner.

There is no known central nervous system cause of this problem. However, it is known that teeth grinding is exacerbated during periods of stress, and jaw tension is a feature of generalized anxiety disorder. Involuntary teeth grinding during the day has been associated with use of recreational drugs, particularly ecstasy. Hence there is ongoing research into the possibility that serotonin or dopamine pathways are involved. Bruxing events during overnight polysomnography are associated with observed lightening of sleep as measured on the electroencephalogram (EEG), suggesting that they are related to anxiety or excess arousal.

Treatment usually includes the use of oral splint appliances to protect the teeth from damage. Cognitive and behavioural interventions, which focus on stress management, lifestyle changes, or improved coping mechanisms, may also be beneficial.

5.1.5 Sleep starts and sleep talking

Sleep starts are muscle jerks that usually occur in light sleep, mostly during the first part of the night. They are common in healthy people and rarely have any adverse consequences. If they are severe or violent, they sometimes wake the subject and they are associated with a sensation of falling. They seem to be most common when there has been marked muscle activity or tension near bedtime in someone who falls asleep rapidly, perhaps because they are very tired (or drunk).

Similarly, talking during sleep is very common in light sleep and rarely has any direct consequences for the patient, but is a source of embarrassment, and can be disturbing to the sleep of the partner.

5.1.6 Head-banging

Head-banging or other rhythmic movements such as rocking are very common in children, but occasionally persist into adulthood. This is not strictly a disorder of non-REM sleep, as it happens at the transition between awake and stage 1 sleep, mostly at the beginning of the night. It is thought that such repetitive movements are a form of comforting, sleep-promoting behaviour, and they are not known to have any direct consequences for the patient. However, in rare cases they can be persistent and lead to disturbing of other sleepers and bruising to the head. Treatment usually consists of explanation and reassurance, and in some cases, protection by pillows or headrests may be required.

5.2 Parasomnias that arise from REM sleep

5.2.1 Nightmares

5.2.1.1 *What are the symptoms of nightmares?*

Almost everyone has experienced nightmares, which are distressing dreams that can have a recurring theme. Most people tolerate them as they are infrequent and relatively undisturbing. However, patients seek help when they occur frequently or cause awakenings. Nightmares differ from night terrors in that when the patient wakes they are oriented, they know that what they have experienced is a bad dream, and they can vividly describe the dream content. It is thought that recalling the dream several times during the day makes it more likely to occur again the following night. In some psychiatric disorders, especially post-traumatic stress disorder (PTSD) and depression, nightmares are more frequent. In PTSD, the nightmares usually involve the reliving of the traumatic incident and can lead to extreme distress. This can be a problem for the bed partner, as when half awake the dreamer may misinterpret them as one of the threatening images in the nightmare and act against them to protect him- or herself. Such PTSD nightmares can occur many years after the incident, and this is thought to be due to the gradual breakdown of cortical inhibitory control of these memories as people age. In depression, nightmares tend to be less person-specific but are often equally frightening, with scenes of doom, disaster, and suffering predominating.

The prevalence of nightmares is unknown, because people who experience nightmares rarely consult health professionals, although this is a key diagnostic symptom in PTSD.

5.2.1.2 *Treatment of nightmares*

Nightmares can be treated effectively with psychological techniques. The best approach is an individual or group programme which includes guided imagery and exposure that attempts to change the imagery from fearful to pleasant content or outcome, and this has been used successfully even in nightmare sufferers with PTSD (Krakow *et al* 2001).

First, the patient is trained to conjure up pleasant imagery, and then they are encouraged to write down a dream and choose a new and non-threatening ending. This process is continued, as they progress to rehearsing the new dream with pleasant imagery. Less severe nightmares have been treated with these methods by providing the patient with postal instructions (Burgess *et al* 1998).

5.2.2 **Sleep paralysis**

5.2.2.1 *What are the symptoms of sleep paralysis?*

- Waking from sleep (which can even be a nap) with a feeling of fear and being unable to move
- Sometimes a feeling of crushing of the chest
- Usually the patient is fully oriented, but sometimes there is persistent imagery from a dream (e.g. of being chased and wanting to scream)
- Sometimes an awareness of an 'ominous presence' nearby

5.2.2.2 *How common is sleep paralysis?*

This disorder can be isolated or it may be associated with narcolepsy. The lifetime prevalence of isolated sleep paralysis has been estimated to be 3%. This increases to about 20% in anxiety disorders (generalized anxiety disorder, panic, and social phobia) (Otto *et al* 2006) and 59% in African Americans with panic disorder (Paradis and Friedman 2005). In the latter study, sleep paralysis was present in 23% of African-American community volunteers and 6% of white community volunteers. In informal polls of audiences at scientific meetings, we have estimated that around 25–30% have had at least one episode.

5.2.2.3 *What causes sleep paralysis?*

The cause is unknown, but the mechanism is an intrusion of the atonia, or paralysis of skeletal muscles, of REM sleep when the person is awake. This usually occurs after a REM episode towards the end of the night, as the person is waking up. The feeling of paralysis is very frightening, and can be made worse if the dream imagery from REM accompanies it. The crushing feeling in the chest may be because the intercostal accessory muscles of respiration, which are needed to take a terrified gasp, are paralysed during REM, but the diaphragm is not.

This feeling of fear, crushing, and an ominous presence is attributed in some cultures to an evil (usually female) being, called an 'old hag' or ghost. Indeed, the term nightmare was first used in the English language to mean a sensation of a heavy, female presence (mare) crushing the body in the night, and probably referred to sleep paralysis.

Episodes of sleep paralysis are more likely to occur when the sleep pattern is disrupted, particularly by sleep loss or irregular timing—for example, shift work or when woken in the middle of the night. Alcohol consumption seems to make it more likely, perhaps because of the withdrawal effects. Typically, the first episode occurs during daytime recovery sleep after staying up all night at a party or on night duty—the term 'night nurse paralysis' has been used for this disorder and illustrates the latter.

5.2.2.4 *Treatment of sleep paralysis*

Improved sleep habits (including reduced alcohol consumption) and reassurance often reduce the frequency of occurrence. Treatment of those with panic disorder with selective serotonin reuptake inhibitors (SSRIs) often does not stop the night-time paralysis. In some individuals, a vicious cycle of alcohol dependence develops where the fear of paralysis lead to onset insomnia, which they overcome by self-medication with alcohol. However, this may lead to more paralysis and more anxiety about sleep, so alcohol intake is increased to a point where dependence, withdrawal, and liver damage ensue.

The episodes of paralysis are terminated immediately when there is sensory input from the limbs; the resulting message from the ascending arousal system 'unlocks' the paralysis. Sometimes the sufferer is able to signal to their bed partner by tiny movements or vocalizations, and some partners have learned to recognize these and touch their partner's arm to end the episode.

There is no known pharmacological treatment for sleep paralysis.

5.2.3 **REM behaviour disorder (RBD)**

5.2.3.1 *What are the symptoms of RBD?*

- Violent, short-duration complex behaviour at night
- Often several episodes per night
- These episodes can wake the subject
- The subject remembers the dream
- Dreams are very vivid, violent, and unpleasant

This disorder is typically characterized by episodes of shouting and a very sudden, violent movement. This could involve grasping an object and lashing out blindly with it, grasping the bed partner violently (sometimes by the neck), punching, etc. There is no awareness of the surroundings, so the patient may easily be hurt by falling from their bed or knocking against furniture. Then they often wake up, become still and confused for a few seconds, and then distressed and remorseful, with recall of a violent dream, for example, in which they or someone close to them was being attacked, and they needed to retaliate violently.

5.2.3.2 *How common is RBD?*

RBD is almost exclusively confined to men. It occurs mostly in men over 50 years of age, and there is increasing prevalence with age.

A very important feature of this disorder is its association with present or future Parkinson's disease and Lewy body dementia. The risk of developing these diseases in patients with RBD is variously assessed at 45–85%, depending on the duration of follow-up.

Its prevalence in the general population is unknown. A telephone survey of 4900 people aged 15–100 years gave an estimated prevalence of RBD of 0.5% (Ohayon *et al* 1997). In another study, involving a community sample of 1034 elderly people, 0.8% reported a history of sleep-related injury. These had physical and psychiatric assessment and a sleep recording, and four people were confirmed to have RBD, giving an estimated prevalence of RBD of 0.38%.

5.2.3.3 *How is RBD diagnosed and treated?*

The diagnosis is usually made with polysomnography, preferably with video recording as well, which shows lack of atonia during REM, and often an episode is recorded, because they tend to be frequent. This lack of atonia or paralysis in REM allows the person to move in response to dreams (most usually frightening nightmares), with consequent risks to self and others.

Antidepressants, particularly SSRIs, tricyclics, and mixed reuptake inhibitors such as venlafaxine, make RBD worse. Bupropion may not have this effect, but the evidence is only anecdotal so far.

Making the sleep environment as safe as possible is the main priority. Sometimes couples have elected to sleep separately, but often a separate bed in the same room is preferred to sleeping in the spare room. RBD is difficult to treat with medication, and there are no controlled trials, but there have been some reports that clonazepam is effective, although it has daytime sedation effects and may exacerbate breathing problems at night. Other case reports and small series have shown some benefit from agomelatine, melatonin, pramipexole, and clonidine.

5.3 **Parasomnias: general points**

- Almost all parasomnias are exacerbated by anxiety, so the patient should 'wind down' in a relaxed and quiet fashion before going to bed.
- There is a high incidence of comorbid anxiety or depressive disorder.
- The incidence of parasomnia is four times higher in patients with obstructive sleep apnoea and in children who snore.
- In snorers, parasomnias follow respiratory events.

Anxiety is increased by:

- fear of injury to self or bed partner
- feeling 'out of control' of one's actions
- the perception that relatives, friends, or professionals 'do not take it seriously.'

Fear of having a parasomnia may lead to onset insomnia.

References

Burgess M, Gill M, Marks I (1998). Postal self-exposure treatment of recurrent nightmares. Randomised controlled trial. *Br J Psychiatry* **172**: 257–62.

Krakow B, Hollifield M, Johnston L *et al* (2001). Imagery rehearsal therapy for chronic nightmares in sexual assault survivors with posttraumatic stress disorder: a randomized controlled trial. *JAMA* **286**: 537–45.

Ohayon MM, Caulet M, Priest RG (1997). Violent behavior during sleep. *J Clin Psychiatry* **58**: 369–76.

Otto MW, Simon NM, Powers M, Hinton D, Zalta AK, Pollack MH (2006). Rates of isolated sleep paralysis in outpatients with anxiety disorders. *J Anxiety Disord* **20**: 687–93.

Paradis CM, Friedman S (2005). Sleep paralysis in African Americans with panic disorder. *Transcult Psychiatry* **42**: 123–34.

Schenck C, Mahowald M (1996). Long-term, nightly benzodiazepine treatment of injurious parasomnias and other disorders of disrupted nocturnal sleep in 170 adults. *Am J Med* **100**: 333–7.

Wilson SJ, Lillywhite AR, Potokar JP, Bell CJ, Nutt DJ (1997). Adult night terrors and paroxetine. *Lancet* **350**: 185.

Chapter 6

Circadian rhythm sleep disorders

Key points

- Circadian rhythm sleep disorders (CRSDs) are disturbances of the normal sleep–wake rhythm, and subtypes include jet lag, delayed sleep phase syndrome (DSPS), advanced sleep phase syndrome (ASPS), irregular sleep–wake rhythm, and shift-work sleep disorder (SWSD)
- Jet lag is the most common circadian rhythm disorder, and is caused by a disturbance of internal circadian rhythm due to rapid travel across multiple time zones
- Recovery from jet lag can be aided by behavioural modification. Pharmacological approaches such as melatonin can also help to alleviate symptoms
- DSPS is more prevalent in adolescents and young adults; ASPS is a much rarer condition than DSPS, and is seen primarily in middle-aged and older adults
- Patients with shift-work sleep disorder often present in middle age after years of trouble-free working

In humans, the sleep–wake rhythm follows a roughly 24-h pattern from day to day. However, if people are kept in constant conditions of dim light with a stable routine, the innate sleep–wake rhythm repeats approximately every 24.2–24.9 h. In the real world, zeitgebers (time-givers), which are stimuli from the external environment, synchronize the internal rhythm to match the 24-h day. The primary zeitgeber is light, but eating, drinking, and regular daily periods of activity such as work also synchronize the rhythm. Light is sensed by specialized receptors in the retina (unrelated to vision) which relay to the suprachiasmatic nuclei (SCN) in the hypothalamus, which orchestrates the body's circadian rhythms. The length of our innate rhythm seems to be genetically determined. For instance, hamsters with a circadian cycle ranging from 20 to 25 h have been bred, and transplanting the SCN from one to the other will change the time of the rhythm in the recipient to that of the donor (Ralph *et al* 1990). Genetic variants that affect circadian rhythms in humans have also been identified (Ebisawa 2007). However, how readily we respond to zeitgebers depends on other factors, such as motivation and genetic influences.

In addition to the length of the internal rhythm, another feature that differs from one person to another is the preferred sleeping time, or chronotype. Some people prefer to go to bed late and wake late, and others prefer to go to bed early and wake early. Chronotype can be assessed with a simple questionnaire asking about sleep and wake times on work days and on free days. The measure that is used in studies of chronotype is the preferred midpoint of sleep, which averages about 4.30 a.m. in adults. This preference is normally distributed over the population, with the two extremes being called 'owls' (preferred midpoint is 2–3 h later, so they go to bed late) and 'larks' (preferred midpoint is 2–3 h earlier, so they go to bed earlier).

Chronotype changes with age. Children have an early midpoint, and then there is a steady increase to about 5.00 a.m. at the end of adolescence (i.e. preferring to go to bed and wake later), followed by a steady decrease during the rest of life, which helps to explain why older people often rise early in the morning. This increase in the teenage years is greater in males, but the maximum increase is reached earlier in females (Roenneberg et al 2004). This fits well with anecdotal accounts of young males having greater difficulty waking in the morning than young females.

6.1 Circadian rhythm sleep disorders (often called sleep-scheduling disorders)

Circadian rhythm sleep disorders are sleep disorders where there is a mismatch between the circadian rhythm and the required sleep–wake cycle. Thus there can be sleeplessness when trying to sleep at a time not signalled by the internal clock, and excessive sleepiness when the person needs to be awake.

Some circadian disorders are due to an individual lifestyle, including work and travel schedules, that conflicts with the internal clock, such as jet lag and shift-work sleep disorder. Others are likely to be innate.

6.1.1 Jet lag

The most common circadian rhythm disorder is jet lag, which is transient and is the result of the internal circadian rhythm being temporarily out of synchronization with the external environment because of rapid travel across time zones.

The symptoms of jet lag are usually daytime fatigue and sleepiness, night-time insomnia, mood changes, difficulty concentrating, general malaise, and stomach upsets. Sudden episodes of feeling hot and sweaty can occur and may be associated with unsteadiness. For most people, jet lag is worse during eastward travel, because our internal rhythm is slightly longer than 24 h, so lengthening the day after westward travel is somewhat easier.

After travel from west to east, difficulty falling asleep is the main sleep problem, and after travel from east to west, early waking is more evident. Symptoms are transient and should resolve as the circadian clock re-establishes synchronization with local time. The rate of adaptation is roughly 1 day per hour of time difference, so after travelling from the US east coast to the UK, resynchronization should take about 5 days.

The recovery process from jet lag can be made easier by a few simple stratagems. On arrival at the end destination, it is important to try to adjust to local time, to eat meals when the locals do, exercise, and generally keep to a routine. Also, it is a good idea to keep awake while it is daytime at the destination. Bright light at appropriate times—for example, in the morning, moving from east to west—and dim light at others (by staying indoors or wearing sunglasses!) can help to speed up adaptation. When the phase change is more than 10 h, it can be difficult to know whether to try to synchronize one's rhythm backwards or forwards, and trial and error is the best method.

Pharmacological approaches can be helpful. Melatonin may help jet lag symptoms if taken in doses of 0.5–5 mg close to local bedtime for up to 4 days (Herxheimer and Petrie 2002). The short-term use of short-acting hypnotic medications such as zolpidem can be useful for alleviating symptoms of insomnia, and caffeine can improve daytime alertness.

6.1.2 Shift-work sleep disorder (SWSD)

There are many people who happily adapt to the demands of working exclusively at night or on rotating shifts, but some experience insomnia when trying to sleep after a night or even evening shift, or on their days off. Others may experience excessive sleepiness when required to be awake on the job. Together, these symptoms lead to a condition called shift-work sleep disorder.

The ability to adapt to changes in sleep–wake routines decreases with age. Patients with shift-work sleep disorder often present in middle age after years of trouble-free working, having now found themselves increasingly unable to cope with the required routine. The disorder is commonly seen in police and nursing staff for whom night work is necessary, and it can be exacerbated by changing family circumstances or changes in the frequency of rotation of shift. The shift that is most difficult to cope with is usually the early one, starting work at 6 or 7 a.m. This is for two reasons. First, going to sleep earlier the night before, in anticipation of an early shift, is generally more difficult, because of the 'forbidden zone' in mid-evening (see Chapter 1). Secondly, on later shifts, people have time to take a nap before work to reduce their sleep debt, but there is no opportunity for this before the early shift.

6.1.2.1 *What are the symptoms of SWSD?*

- Unrefreshing sleep
- Excessive sleepiness when one is required to be awake
- Insomnia when one is not working
- Sleep deprivation may lead to impaired performance at work or on driving home
- The symptoms may persist on days off

6.1.2.2 *How common is SWSD?*

Recent figures suggest that for 25% of people their working hours are outside the standard 9 a.m. to 5 p.m. working day, and up to 10% of these individuals may have shift-work sleep disorder, so the problem is likely to be huge. However, relatively few sufferers or doctors are aware of it, so presentation for help is rare unless the person's work or career comes under threat or lives are put at risk—for example, by police personnel falling asleep when driving at work.

6.1.2.3 *What is the cause of SWSD?*

The cause is failure to adjust the internal clock to the work schedule, so that working is demanded when the internal clock (and sometimes homeostatic processes, too) are signalling that it is time to be asleep, and conversely sleep is demanded when waking processes are high.

6.1.2.4 *How do we diagnose and treat SWSD?*

A full history and a diary for several shift cycles may be sufficient, but sometimes actigraphy will reveal information about nap timing, which can be used as a basis for advice. Careful elucidation of other factors, such as drug and alcohol use, depression, and other sleep disorders (e.g. sleep apnoea, movement disorders) is essential.

There are two main treatment goals. The first is to try to synchronize the internal clock with the work schedule, and this is most likely to succeed in people with fixed shifts. A regular sleep–wake routine, bright light in the desired 'daytime', and darkness at sleep times, together with sensible use of caffeine and alcohol, are the main approaches. Bedtimes should be protected and long enough for adequate sleep. Of course, for this regime to work properly, it must be maintained at weekends and during rest periods, which is often unacceptable for family and social reasons. In extreme cases, this disorder is a justification for redeployment from a job that requires shift attendance, and this usually rectifies the problem. More advice can be found in Chapter 10.

6.1.3 **Delayed sleep phase syndrome (DSPS)**

DSPS means that sleep times are delayed relative to the desired or socially acceptable schedule.

6.1.3.1 *What are the symptoms of DSPS?*

- Difficulty falling asleep before 2–3 a.m. (sometimes later)
- On weekends or days without work/school/college, the preferred waking time is after 10 a.m.
- Sleep-onset insomnia and difficulty waking up in the morning on days when the person needs to work, say, 9 a.m. to 5 p.m.

Therefore these patients have symptoms of both insomnia and hypersomnia, and either or both of these are causing problems with daytime function.

6.1.3.2 *How common is DSPS?*

The prevalence of DSPS in the general population is 0.1–0.2%, and perhaps about 10% in adolescents and young adults.

A common presentation is a university student who has early lectures or seminars perhaps once or twice a week, and tends to fall asleep in these. The nights before these lectures, they try to go to bed early but remain awake for hours. On other nights, they will socialize, use the computer to work or surf the Internet, or play video games, all of which mean that they will be experiencing both internal arousal and well-lit conditions late in the evening. Both of these promote wakefulness, delaying sleep further. The student is distressed by the insomnia and is having great difficulty with keeping up with their academic work.

An actigraph recording from one such case is shown in Figure 6.1.

6.1.3.3 *What is the cause of DSPS?*

There is likely to be a combination of genetic and environmental factors. There is evidence that certain polymorphisms in the circadian rhythm genes (e.g. period [per]) are more common in individuals with DSPS. This may result in a relative insensitivity to

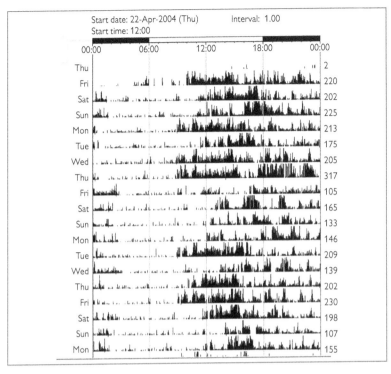

Start date: 22-Apr-2004 (Thu)   Interval: 1.00
Start time: 12:00

	00:00	06:00	12:00	18:00	00:00	
Thu						2
Fri						220
Sat						202
Sun						225
Mon						213
Tue						175
Wed						205
Thu						317
Fri						105
Sat						165
Sun						133
Mon						146
Tue						209
Wed						139
Thu						202
Fri						230
Sat						198
Sun						107
Mon						155

Figure 6.1 Actigraph recording from a young man with delayed sleep phase syndrome and an irregular routine. The periods of relatively low activity (sleep) vary in time placement. On most days they begin between 1 a.m. and 3 a.m. and end between 11 a.m. and 12 noon. On some days, however, the subject has college commitments in the morning and rises at 9 a.m.

zeitgebers. Environmental and behavioural factors such as reduced exposure to light during the early morning (due to sleeping in) and prolonged exposure to light later in the evening (see Section 6.1.3) will contribute to and perpetuate the delayed pattern. Also, there may be a disruption in homeostatic sleep mechanisms, as some studies have shown that people with DSPS have poorer recovery sleep after sleep deprivation.

6.1.3.4 How is DSPS diagnosed and treated?

It is important to establish whether or not delayed sleep schedules are causing significant daytime impairment or distress. Although the diagnosis is made primarily by the patient's history, keeping a sleep diary for at least 2 weeks is essential. Actigraphy is often very useful, and again should be conducted for at least 2 weeks so that the data include the activity from at least two weekends, in order that the sleep–wake pattern can be assessed in the real world and in the absence of time pressures. A psychiatric, drug, and alcohol history is essential to eliminate many other common causes of altered sleep.

Polysomnography is usually normal and is not useful except if there is still doubt about the diagnosis after completion of a diary and actigraphy, and other sleep disorders need to be excluded.

Treatment depends on the severity of the disorder, the potential compliance of the patient, and their work or school obligations. One of the most effective treatments is timed bright light exposure. The best light is daylight, and there should be strict adherence to a routine that involves getting up at an agreed time, say 8 a.m., and being outside or near a window for at least an hour. In addition, there should be a policy of living with dim light in the hours near to the desired bedtime. With other elements of good sleep habits, such as careful use of caffeine and alcohol, avoidance of daytime napping, and reduction of arousing activities (e.g. computer games in the evening), there should be an improvement in sleep and alertness after 2 weeks.

Chronotherapy is another approach, which involves the circadian clock being reset by gradually delaying sleep and wake times by 1–2 h each day until the desired sleep and wake times are reached. This is very demanding and difficult in individuals with work or family commitments, but is effective in motivated patients. An alternative approach is to use melatonin, which has been shown to be effective when taken at doses of up to 3 mg at the desired bedtime; this is a useful option when light therapy is not possible.

These patients often have an enduring tendency to the disorder, and need to be counselled that they may slip back into the delayed pattern, so treatment may be needed again in the future. DSPS can have a major impact on life and work, and patients often need to think carefully about the type of life they lead and the jobs they do. Careers that are not suitable for people with this tendency include shift work and on-call work (e.g. medicine) or other occupations that involve changing time zones (e.g. the aviation industry). Patients often choose jobs where late bedtimes are the norm (e.g. in a restaurant or in the entertainment business).

6.1.4 Advanced sleep phase syndrome (ASPS)

This is a much less common disorder, and is rarely seen in the young.

6.1.4.1 *What are the symptoms of ASPS?*

- Habitual sleep and wake times 2–3 h earlier than desired
- Sleep maintenance insomnia
- Early-morning awakenings
- Sleepiness in the late afternoon or early evening

6.1.4.2 *How common is ASPS?*

Young people rarely have this disorder, but it occurs in about 1% of middle-aged and older adults.

6.1.4.3 *What is the cause of ASPS?*

As for DSPS, the cause of ASPS is unknown, but genetic factors are involved. Families with this disorder have been reported, and there are some mutations in clock genes in these. It is thought that people who have a short circadian rhythm or are less responsive to light cues are more likely to suffer from ASPS.

6.1.3.4 *How is ASPS diagnosed and treated?*

Sleep history, sleep diaries, and perhaps actigraphy will help to make the diagnosis. Again other disorders should be excluded, particularly depression, because early-morning waking may indicate this.

Treatment with bright light in the evening, thereby delaying sleep, may also delay awakening and so improve sleep. There is little evidence for the use of melatonin or hypnotics; if the latter were tried, then hypnotics with a moderate half-life (e.g. temazepam, zopiclone) would be the most suitable, as sleep prolongation is the goal.

6.1.5 **Non-24-hour circadian rhythm disorder (free running)**

6.1.5.1 *What are the symptoms?*

The key diagnostic feature is that of a daily increment of sleep and wake times (getting later each day). This is often associated with insomnia of varying severity, and daytime sleepiness.

Patients usually try to keep to a regular pattern, which is satisfactory when the internal rhythm is in phase with the world, and on the few days when they are roughly synchronized their sleep can be normal. However, when the internal rhythm is out of phase with conventional sleep and wake times the symptoms will be worse.

6.1.5.2 *How common is free running?*

This condition is rare in sighted people but is very much more common in those with total blindness (e.g. from birth). Some studies have shown that up to 50% of totally blind people have these free-running rhythms and chronic sleep disturbances.

6.1.5.3 *What causes free running?*

The most likely cause is reduced light perception, so that the internal circadian rhythm is not synchronized to the 24-h day. Not all blind people have these problems, and this could be explained by the preservation of the melanopsin receptors in the eye, which can signal to the hypothalamic clock independently of vision. Melanopsin is a recently discovered photopigment that plays a primary role in regulating circadian rhythms in mice, where knocking out the gene that makes it leads to a free-running animal that is insensitive to light entrainment. Melanopsin is found in the human eye and is believed to play a similar role, although research into demonstrating this has only just begun. Even if blind people have no means of light input to the circadian brain system, other zeitgebers such as work routine and physical activity can sometimes provide sufficient stimulus to the clock to keep it synchronized.

6.1.5.4 *How do we diagnose and treat free running?*

Again sleep diaries and actigraphy are useful, and both of these should be continued for about 4 weeks to see the true pattern of daily drift (see Figure 6.2).

Treatment is by rigid attention to daily routine of sleep times and physical activities and to other aspects of good sleep habits. In blind people, this is usually combined with melatonin (2–4 mg) administered at bedtime. However, in those few patients who are sighted, maintaining regular morning daylight exposure is likely to be a much stronger stimulus to the clock than melatonin.

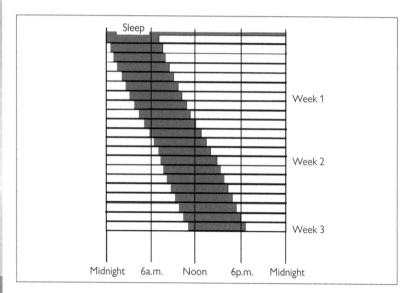

Figure 6.2 Illustration of free-running sleep–wake rhythm. The dark sections represent sleep, and the sleep periods move gradually through the day over a period of weeks. Night-time placement of high sleep propensity occurs every 5–6 weeks.

6.1.6 **Irregular sleep–wake rhythm**

- Sleep periods occur irregularly from day to day.
- There may be napping between longer periods of sleep.

This disorder occurs in dementia and in people with brain damage such as in learning disability, and more recently has been described in some people with schizophrenia (Wulff *et al* 2011). It may reflect central deficits in clock mechanisms or decreased responsiveness of the system. Melatonin secretion becomes more fragmented in these individuals, probably as the progressive neuronal loss affects the SCN. However, irregular sleep–wake rhythm is also encountered in people who voluntarily maintain irregular sleep–wake routines.

Treatment is primarily behaviourally based, with an emphasis on increasing interesting daytime activities, maximizing exposure to ambient light, especially in the mornings, and keeping to strict bedtimes. These bedtimes should be tailored to the overall amount of sleep that the patient usually experiences over 24 h. This is often very difficult and demanding for carers, but has been shown to be effective in improving sleep consolidation at night. There is a small amount of evidence that melatonin may improve sleep–wake patterns in children with learning disability, but the evidence in dementia is not consistent.

For further information on genetic discoveries in these circadian disorders, see Hida *et al* (2012), and for recommendations for treatment see the British Association for

Psychopharmacology (BAP) consensus statement at <www.bap.org.uk/pdfs/bap_sleep_guidelines.pdf>.

References

Ebisawa T (2007). Circadian rhythms in the CNS and peripheral clock disorders: human sleep disorders and clock genes. *J Pharmacol Sci* **103**: 150–54.

Herxheimer A, Petrie KJ (2002). Melatonin for the prevention and treatment of jet lag. *Cochrane Database Syst Rev* **2**: CD001520.

Hida A, Kitamura S, Mishima K (2012). Pathophysiology and pathogenesis of circadian rhythm sleep disorders. *J Physiol Anthropol* **31**: 7.

Ralph MR, Foster RG, Davis FC, Menaker M (1990). Transplanted suprachiasmatic nucleus determines circadian period. *Science* **247**: 975–8.

Roenneberg T, Kuehnle T, Pramstaller PP *et al* (2004). A marker for the end of adolescence. *Curr Biol* **14**: R1038–9.

Wulff K, Dijk DJ, Middleton B, Foster RG, Joyce E (2011). Sleep and circadian rhythm disruption in schizophrenia patients. *Br J Psychiatry* **200**: 308–16.

Chapter 7

Psychiatric disorders and sleep

Key points

- Sleep problems are common in patients with psychiatric conditions, including depression, anxiety (post-traumatic stress disorder, generalized anxiety disorder, and panic disorder), bipolar disorder, schizophrenia, dementia, and substance abuse
- Insomnia is the most common sleep complaint related to psychiatric disorders; it can worsen the prognosis in mania and depression, and can signal an imminent relapse
- Sleep problems and depression are strongly linked; about 75% of depressed patients have a major sleep complaint, and short REM latency, decreased slow-wave sleep, and increased wakefulness are present in 40–70% of depressed outpatients
- The ability of antidepressant drugs to improve sleep early in treatment is often important to patients, particularly if insomnia causes significant distress
- 5HT2-blocking drugs can improve subjective sleep quickly in depression; tricyclic antidepressants can also do this, but have more unwanted side effects
- Worsening of symptoms in the late afternoon and evening in dementia ('sundowning') is a common problem

Sleep disorders are common in many psychiatric disorders, with the most commonly reported sleep problem in most cases being insomnia. In mania, and possibly in depression, insomnia can significantly worsen the disorder, and early intervention to improve sleep may help to abort a relapse. Also, insomnia is often a prodromal warning sign of imminent relapse. In addition to increased insomnia, there can also be an increased incidence of parasomnias, circadian rhythm disorders, and hypersomnia. For these reasons, enquiring about sleep should be a routine part of patient assessment in psychiatry (see Box 7.1).

7.1 Depression

Sleep difficulties are among the most common symptoms in depressed patients (see Table 7.1). Insomnia is often the reason why depressed patients seek help, and relief of sleep disturbance may encourage compliance with antidepressant treatment. Apart

- **Depression**
  Highest incidence, about 75% have insomnia—improves as mood lifts
  5–10% have hypersomnia—associated with atypical depression
- **Post-traumatic stress disorder**
  Insomnia
  Parasomnias—nightmares, night terrors, sleepwalking
- **Generalized anxiety disorder**
  Insomnia (onset), about 20–30%
- **Panic disorder**
  Nocturnal panic attacks
  Sometimes onset insomnia when fearing these attacks
- **Schizophrenia**
  Insomnia (onset and maintenance)—incidence unknown
  Scheduling disorder ('free running')
- **Dementias**
  Insomnia
  Agitation at bedtime/'sundowning'
  Scheduling disorder (sleep in daytime)
- **Withdrawal from opiates or alcohol**
  Insomnia is common
  High risk factor for relapse
  Irregular or chaotic sleep–wake scheduling

Table 7.1 Sleep and depression are strongly linked	
• Insomnia is common in depression—it may be the presenting complaint	• Sleep architecture is abnormal in depression
• Sleep disturbance may predict treatment outcome	• Antidepressants change sleep architecture in the opposite direction
• Sleep manipulation alters mood	

from the discomfort that sleep problems produce, they may lead to exhaustion, poor functioning during the day, and accidents, and they are associated with an increase in suicide risk.

About 75% of depressed patients complain of at least one of the following: difficulty falling asleep, fragmented sleep, disturbing dreams, early-morning wakening, decreased amount of sleep, not feeling refreshed in the morning, and feeling tired during the day. A minority of patients sleep excessively during their illness, especially those with bipolar or atypical depression.

Objectively, sleep architecture is disturbed in depression with changes in rapid eye movement (REM) onset latency and in the distribution of slow-wave sleep (SWS). These changes constitute some of the most robust biological findings in depression, and they have been studied for years as potential indicators of response to treatment and relapse, as well as giving pointers to the underlying neurochemical abnormalities. There is no exact agreement between what is reported subjectively and what is found in objective assessments of sleep of depressed patients, so both approaches are used in the evaluation of patients, especially in research settings, and they provide useful information that can be used clinically.

Sleep disorders in depression have predictive value, because there is evidence in recurrent depression that psychological therapies may be less effective in patients with abnormal sleep architecture (Thase *et al* 1996).

7.1.1 Objective sleep changes in depression

Polysomnographic studies of depression have confirmed a number of signs of sleep disturbance in this condition (Benca *et al* 1992).

- Compared with normal controls, sleep continuity of depressed subjects is often impaired, with increased wakefulness and reduced sleep efficiency.
- Sleep onset latency is significantly increased, and total sleep time is reduced.
- SWS may be reduced. In particular the normal pattern of slow-wave activity decreasing from the first to the last non-REM (NREM) episode (see Chapter 1) is disrupted, with most SWS occurring in the second episode in depressed patients.
- REM latency is often shortened, and the duration of the first REM period is increased.
- The number of eye movements in REM may also be increased.

These changes indicate that, in depression, there is disruption of both the circadian and the homeostatic aspects of sleep. Short REM latency, decreased SWS, and increased wakefulness are present in 40–70% of depressed outpatients. These changes are illustrated in the hypnogram of a depressed patient in Figure 7.1.

7.1.2 Effects of antidepressant treatment on sleep of depressed patients

From the clinical point of view, the subjective perception of sleep is more important than polysomnographic findings. In general, in most of the studies of sleep complaints during antidepressant treatment, the comparator is sleep at baseline, and there is improvement over a period of weeks as the depression lifts. This is seen with both drug and cognitive therapies. Differences between drugs have been reported early in treatment, but these differences are generally much smaller or absent after 2–6 weeks (Wilson and Argyropoulos 2005).

However, the ability of different drugs to improve sleep early in treatment is often important to patients, particularly if insomnia is causing significant distress. Also, early improvement of sleep symptoms may encourage the patient to carry on with medication to the point where the mood-lifting effects become apparent (usually within 2–3 weeks).

Antidepressants that are 5HT2 blockers, such as mirtazapine and agomelatine (a 5HT2 antagonist and melatonin-receptor agonist), can improve subjective sleep quickly in depression. Tricyclic antidepressants (TCAs) such as trimipramine and

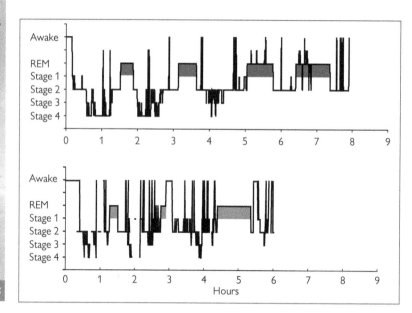

Figure 7.1 Hypnograms showing a normal subject (upper) and a depressed patient (lower). REM episodes are shown as darker bars. Time to REM onset (REM onset latency) in the normal subject is 80 min, and in the depressed patient is about 60 min. The patient has many awakenings during sleep and wakes early in the morning.

doxepin also do this, because they are potent histamine H1 antagonists, but have more unwanted side effects such as carry-over sedation and dry mouth.

Objectively, SSRIs, alerting TCAs, and mixed uptake blocker antidepressants decrease REM sleep and REM latency (see Figure 7.2), but can increase waking in sleep early in treatment, for which a hypnotic is sometimes required. Mirtazapine, mianserin, trazodone, and trimipramine have smaller effects on REM, but decrease waking in sleep in the first weeks of treatment.

SWS tends to increase overall after chronic treatment in depression, and this may be either a general effect of sleep improvement or related to resolution of the biological processes that lead to depression. However, there is evidence that the imbalance of SWS mentioned earlier may be a trait of depressed patients.

7.1.2.1 Sleep deprivation as an intervention in depression

Somewhat paradoxically, total sleep deprivation has been known for many years to improve mood the next day in major depression. This is an extension of the feature observed in many patients with severe depression that their mood is worse in the morning and gradually improves during the day, so it can be in the normal range just before bed, only to revert during sleep. However, it is difficult to keep patients awake all night, and once they are allowed uninterrupted sleep, all of the beneficial effects disappear. Some research has refined the methods of manipulation of sleep and circadian

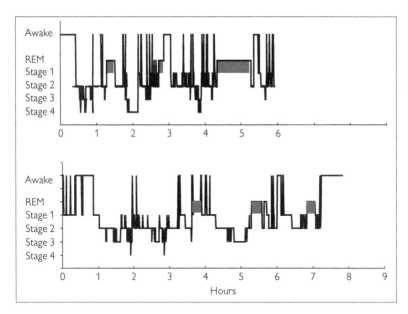

Figure 7.2 The same depressed patient before (upper) and after (lower) 3 days of treatment with the selective serotonin reuptake inhibitor (SSRI) paroxetine. REM latency has increased to 165 min, and the REM amount is decreased. Waking occurs later in the morning. There are many episodes of lightening of sleep to stage 1.

rhythm to maximize its effects on mood by bringing the sleep period forward, and several strategies have been proposed to prolong the therapeutic effect, such as adding drug interventions and strictly controlling the amount and type of sleep allowed in the following days (Giedke 2004).

7.2 Bipolar disorder

Sleep in bipolar disorder is state dependent, with a manic phase usually being preceded by a shortened duration of sleep—this can be a useful early warning.

Some patients also have longer duration of sleep and an increased amount of day-time sleepiness during a depressed phase.

Objective sleep changes are similar to those in unipolar depression.

7.3 Generalized anxiety disorder

Sleep onset insomnia is experienced by around 20–30% of patients with generalized anxiety disorder (GAD), and sometimes sleep is the main focus of anxiety. They may also have increased night-time awakenings and report poor sleep quality. There are few objective abnormalities apart from reduced sleep continuity. Some authors believe that primary insomnia is a variant of GAD, where the main focus of the worry is on sleep and the negative consequences of having too little of it. Patients may spend hours ruminating before sleep onset, and this is sometimes ameliorated by treatment with SSRIs, even though in depression these drugs can often disrupt sleep early in treatment. The newer anxiolytic, pregabalin, has modest effects in improving sleep.

In large clinical trials, it has been shown that sleep improves along with other symptoms after effective antidepressant treatment. Cognitive behavioural therapy (CBT) focusing on sleep also appears to be efficacious in this group, similar to its actions in patients with primary insomnia (see Chapter 3).

7.4 Post-traumatic stress disorder (PTSD)

There is a high incidence of almost all sleep disorders in PTSD. Around 70–90% of patients with PTSD have difficulty falling asleep or staying asleep, and nightmares are reported by 20–70%. Parasomnias such as sleepwalking and night terrors are more common than in the general population, and more recently a high incidence of sleep-disordered breathing and sleep movement disorders has also been reported.

In a study of car accident survivors, sleep complaints at 1 month after the trauma were higher in the group who had PTSD a year later, so there may be some predictive value in assessing sleep (Koren *et al* 2002).

Objective measures of sleep disturbance are inconsistent, but most studies show decreased sleep efficiency. There is controversy about REM sleep, with some reports of REM decreases and other reports of increases. However, there does seem to be a consistent trend towards more awakenings during REM episodes, and this together with the reduced sleep efficiency appears to indicate hyperarousal at night.

Drug therapy used for PTSD symptoms, such as SSRIs, trazodone, and mirtazapine, may improve sleep and nightmares. More recently, there have been encouraging reports of sleep improvements after treatment with prazosin, a centrally acting α1-adrenoceptor antagonist, and also with buspirone, gabapentin, and tiagabine, which need to be confirmed. Evidence suggests that benzodiazepines, TCAs, and monoamine oxidase inhibitors (MAOIs) are not useful for the treatment of PTSD-related sleep disorders.

Cognitive behavioural interventions that target insomnia and imagery rehearsal therapy for nightmares (see Chapter 5) have also demonstrated good outcomes.

7.5 Panic disorder

There are no specific associations between panic disorder and sleep disorders except in those patients who experience night-time panic attacks. Up to 50% of panic disorder patients have at least one of these nocturnal panic attacks, and 30% experience them regularly. In this group, fear of falling asleep becomes a problem, and they describe onset insomnia.

Nocturnal panic attacks do not differ in characteristics from the daytime attacks in a particular patient. When they have occurred during polysomnography, they usually follow a sudden awakening at the transition between stage 2 and stage 3 sleep—that is, just as the patient is descending into deep sleep. They are usually vividly recalled.

Anecdotally, we have seen several patients who have described panic attacks right at the onset of sleep, and in these patients there has been a very high degree of physical awareness of heart rate and/or respiration. In healthy people, there is a slowing of heart rate and a short period of very shallow respiration at sleep onset as the autonomic system resets to its 'sleep' settings. It may be that these patients are abnormally aware of these changes, or that their innate alarm system to carbon dioxide alterations is abnormal, so that the small increase in carbon dioxide levels that occurs in the transition activates the brainstem sensors in vulnerable patients, and these provoke a panic attack.

Apart from the nights with panic attacks, patients with panic disorder do not show any differences in sleep architecture from healthy controls.

7.6 Schizophrenia

Patients with schizophrenia can suffer from insomnia, which is mostly described at times of acute symptoms. They can also experience prolonged sleep or excessive napping in the day, and although this is often thought to be due to the adverse effects of sedating antipsychotic medication, there may be other factors that have only recently been identified, especially circadian dysregulation. The disorder that has been most consistently described in schizophrenia is circadian rhythm disorder (Wulff et al 2011), usually of the non-24-h rhythm type, with gradual delay of the sleep period relative to the day. The cause of this is unknown, but it presumably reflects some biological perturbations in the brain such that the sleep–wake routine appears to lose its normal sensitivity to zeitgebers (see Chapter 7), and in some cases a free-running cycle can emerge, which normalizes once the acute relapse is over. Environmental factors may also play a part, because the lifestyle of many patients can lead to them experiencing fewer of these—for example, because they are spending most of the time in dim light indoors or in hospital, not having regular periods of activity, etc. However, it is possible that at times of acute illness these patients are indeed less sensitive to external cues, and this is an area of active research endeavour at present.

Treatment using normal environmental entraining processes, such as light and exercise, can be difficult in these patients, because the motivation to change lifestyle and engage in such programmes is often low. In the patient whose actigraph is shown in Figure 7.3, the rhythm stabilized for the week or so after his depot antipsychotic injections were resumed, but it should be noted that in some reports in the literature this free-running disorder is attributed to antipsychotic medication.

7.7 Dementia

Increasing age in healthy people is associated with increasing amounts of waking during the night, and this characteristic appears to be worse in dementia, so there is often insomnia. More extreme fragmentation of the 24-h sleep–wake pattern with more sleeping in the daytime and less at night is also common and, of course, compounds the issue as daytime naps reduce the S-process drive to sleep at night and poor night-time sleep makes daytime napping more likely. In addition, there is a significant incidence of REM sleep behaviour disorder in patients with dementia with Lewy bodies (see Chapter 5), probably reflecting the important role of dopamine depletion in this form of dementia.

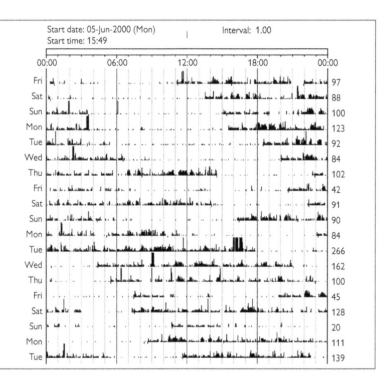

Figure 7.3 Actigraph recording of a schizophrenic patient whose sleep–wake routine was 'free running.' This is a double-plot display and should be compared with that for the normal subject shown in Chapter 2. Note how the inactive (sleep) period runs from 12.30 to 11 a.m. at the top and gets later each day. General levels of activity during the wake period are low.

Treatment of sleep fragmentation and night-time waking should focus on behavioural strategies in the first instance, and where such programmes have been enthusiastically instigated in treatment settings, clear improvements in circadian behaviour have been reported. Boredom and inactivity during the day, especially if associated with reduced or dim levels of light, make daytime napping more likely, and should be avoided as far as possible.

Worsening of symptoms in the late afternoon and evening in dementia ('sundowning') is a common problem, and sometimes the behaviour is very difficult to manage, with confused wandering and occasionally hallucinations in a person who has been much less confused earlier in the day. This is now thought to be due to the progressive damage in cholinergic nuclei such as the nucleus basalis of Meynert that are concerned with arousal, and which are inappropriately activated in these patients when the cortex is programmed to be asleep. The use of bright light in the evening has been reported to help, as has general establishment of good sleep habits, with more activity and less napping during the day. Cholinergic drugs (e.g. donepezil and rivastigmine) may also be of value, as they may rectify the cholinergic dysfunction for a while.

7.8 Substance abuse

7.8.1 Alcohol

In non-dependent drinkers, alcohol promotes sleep, both by shortening the time taken to fall asleep (sleep onset latency) and by increasing deep restorative SWS sleep in the first part of the night, although the pay-off is that later in the night sleep is worse than it would be without alcohol. However, in heavy and dependent daily drinkers the opposite situation occurs, so that sleep is difficult to initiate and is lighter and more interrupted than normal, probably because of changes in brain receptors such as gamma-aminobutyric acid-A (GABA-A) and glutamate. This fragmented pattern persists into abstinence, usually for several weeks, although it will respond to some extent to the usual treatment of withdrawal—that is, long-acting benzodiazepines. However, the use of these drugs to promote sleep in the long term is problematic, as they work in the same way on the GABA-A receptor system as alcohol, which means that they share some subjective experiences like alcohol, and thus can be misused or abused instead of it.

The subjective experience of insomnia, with difficulty getting off to sleep, frequent and prolonged awakenings during the night, and early-morning wakening, is very common in abstinent alcohol-dependent patients. In fact, about 60% of alcohol-dependent patients suffer from insomnia before they stop drinking, and many have probably self-medicated with alcohol in order to get to sleep. Moreover, a high number of alcohol-dependent people are also depressed, and as insomnia is common in depression, the effects of the two conditions are additive.

Sleep problems are not only distressing but also predict relapse in abstinent alcohol-dependent patients. Patients who had insomnia while they were drinking are twice as likely to relapse as those with a normal sleep pattern (Brower *et al* 2001). In addition to these symptoms of insomnia, abstinent alcoholics often have a chaotic lifestyle, which has become established during drinking and takes a long time to settle down to a regular pattern. This results in poor sleep habits and sometimes circadian rhythm disorder, such as the irregular non-24-h pattern shown in Figure 7.4.

7.8.2 Opiate detoxification

During acute opiate withdrawal there are usually severe problems with insomnia. This is probably due to a massive rebound activation of brain arousal systems, especially the noradrenaline projections from the locus coeruleus to the cortex. For reasons that are unclear, but may reflect interactions with other neurotransmitter systems, sleep problems are more prolonged and probably more distressing in people withdrawing from methadone, and there is some evidence that this insomnia is still present at 6 months of abstinence. This is a particular problem as sleep disturbance is a significant factor in predicting relapse, yet is one that has been little studied and is not well understood.

Objectively, there are changes in sleep architecture during opiate detoxification, which are often difficult to interpret because of previous polydrug use, especially of benzodiazepines, alcohol, and cocaine. However, the amount of waking during sleep increases and may remain high for weeks.

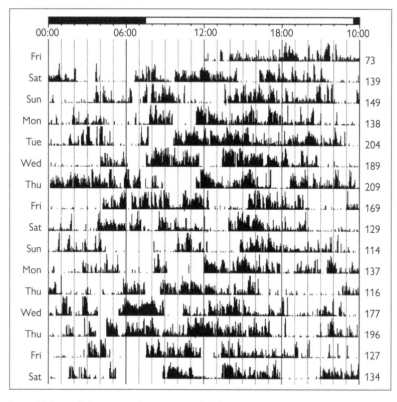

Figure 7.4 Actigraph showing irregular routine in an alcoholic person who had been abstinent for 2 weeks. There are no consistent sleeping and waking times, with naps and short sleeps interspersed with varying levels of waking activity.

7.8.3 Treatment of sleep problems in alcohol and opiate withdrawal

This should focus on cognitive and behavioural strategies to improve sleep habits and reduce anxiety about the consequences of lack of sleep (see Chapter 3). Drug treatment is probably contraindicated, but in alcoholics with depression a more sleep-promoting antidepressant (e.g. mirtazapine, trazodone) would be a sensible choice. In early opiate withdrawal, antihistamines have been used successfully to improve sleep onset insomnia, and often a Z-drug is given for a short period to tide the patient over the worst of the withdrawal; without this form of pharmacological help, many patients will not go through with the withdrawal regime. It is worth noting that the use of α2-adrenoceptor agonists such as clonidine and lofexidine to treat opiate withdrawal may also improve sleep by switching off arousal systems, so these drugs can be given at night as well as in the day.

7.8.4 **Stimulants**

Chronic use of amphetamine and other stimulants is associated with shortened sleep duration and REM suppression, which is due to the direct effects of the drugs releasing dopamine and noradrenaline in the brain. Adaptive homeostatic changes occur in the brain so that during the first 2 weeks of withdrawal there is a rebound of both of these. This leads to the clinical symptoms of daytime sleepiness and fatigue and the nocturnal effects, especially of increased REM sleep, with associated reports of vivid and unpleasant dreaming.

References

Benca RM, Obermeyer WH, Thisted RA, Gillin JC (1992). Sleep and psychiatric disorders: a meta-analysis. *Arch Gen Psychiatry* **49**: 651–70.

Brower KJ, Aldrich MS, Robinson EA, Zucker RA, Greden JF (2001). Insomnia, self-medication, and relapse to alcoholism. *Am J Psychiatry* **158**: 399–404.

Giedke H (2004). The usefulness of therapeutic sleep deprivation in depression. *J Affect Disord* **78**: 85–6.

Koren D, Arnon I, Lavie P, Klein E (2002). Sleep complaints as early predictors of posttraumatic stress disorder: a 1-year prospective study of injured survivors of motor vehicle accidents. *Am J Psychiatry* **159**: 855–7.

Thase ME, Simons AD, Reynolds CF III (1996). Abnormal electroencephalographic sleep profiles in major depression: association with response to cognitive behavior therapy. *Arch Gen Psychiatry* **53**: 99–108.

Wilson S, Argyropoulos S (2005). Antidepressants and sleep: a qualitative review of the literature. *Drugs* **65**: 927–47.

Wulff K, Dijk DJ, Middleton B, Foster RG, Joyce E (2011). Sleep and circadian rhythm disruption in schizophrenia patients. *Br J Psychiatry* **200**: 308–16.

Chapter 8

Sleep disorders associated with neurological and medical disorders

Key points

- Sleep problems are associated with restless legs syndrome (RLS), periodic limb movements disorder (PLMD), Parkinson's disease, and chronic fatigue syndrome
- RLS affects about 4% of men and 5–6% of women, and the incidence increases with age
- Around 80% of patients with RLS also experience periodic leg movements, but only 30% of patients with periodic leg movements have RLS
- Patients with Parkinson's disease experience a variety of sleep complaints, including insomnia, REM sleep behaviour disorder (RBD), excessive day-time sleepiness, and, in some rare cases, sudden sleep attacks

8.1 Restless legs syndrome (RLS)

This is a disorder characterized by an almost irresistible urge to move, usually associated with disagreeable leg sensations, worse during inactivity, and often interfering with sleep.

8.1.1 What are the symptoms of RLS?

- A desire to move the limbs, usually associated with paraesthesia
- Creepy, crawly, tingly feelings, like worms or insects crawling over the skin
- A painful, burning, or aching sensation
- A sensation like water running over the skin
- Sometimes indescribable
- Motor restlessness
- Worse at rest, and partially relieved by activity
- Worse in the evening or at night
- May cause onset insomnia or prolonged night-time awakenings

Patients find that activity temporarily, although only partially, relieves the discomfort, and they sometimes develop stereotyped habits and behaviours that help. The feelings are very much dependent on the time of day, most commonly increasing in intensity during the evening and peaking at or after bedtime. This circadian rhythm of symptoms persists even in people with 'unconventional' sleep–wake cycles.

8.1.2 How common is RLS?

About 4% of men and 5–6% of women suffer from RLS in the population studies, with increasing incidence with age. There is an increased incidence in people with renal disease and in pregnant women. Familial associations have been found, particularly in those whose symptoms start at a young age. Some drugs, notably antidepressants and antihistamines, can precipitate or worsen RLS.

8.1.3 What causes RLS?

The cause is not known, but current theories suggest that there is probably an abnormality in brain dopamine receptor activity, since drugs that increase the function of this neurotransmitter are effective. However, imaging studies of dopamine receptors in the brain have proved inconclusive so far. Abnormalities of iron levels in the brain have been shown in these patients, with a tendency for low levels of this metal in the basal ganglia.

8.1.4 How is RLS diagnosed and treated?

Diagnosis is solely clinical, because it centres on the subjective experience of restlessness (in contrast with periodic limb movement disorder, PLMD; see Section 8.2). Given that this condition is difficult to treat, it is usually managed by neurologists and sleep specialists. Non-pharmacological treatment should include consideration of reducing or stopping medications known to exacerbate RLS, and improving sleep habits if these are noticeably poor. Some patients find that cooling the legs or exercise brings some relief.

The best evidence for drug effectiveness is for drugs that increase dopamine function, such as levodopa and dopamine agonists (Hening *et al* 2004). All of these improve symptoms, but they have each shown varying problems, with the worsening of symptoms of RLS (and PLMD; see Section 8.2) being apparent when the drug is wearing off, known as augmentation. Careful monitoring of the dosage and dose regime is necessary. There is some evidence that the opiates oxycodone and codeine, and the anticonvulsant gabapentin, can also provide some relief.

8.2 Periodic limb movement disorder (PLMD)

8.2.1 What are the symptoms of PLMD?

- Insomnia or excessive sleepiness
- Repetitive highly stereotyped limb movements, which in the leg are characterized by extension of the big toe and flexion of the ankle, knee, and hip
- Movements occur every 20–40 s for periods of minutes or hours
- May be associated with arousals

Periodic limb movements, especially in the legs, can occur in many healthy people, and cause no ill effects apart from kicking the bed partner. They occur in bouts during the night, mostly in light stage 2 sleep. If they cause arousals from sleep, there may be associated insomnia and daytime sleepiness due to sleep fragmentation. Only then is this considered to be a sleep disorder.

8.2.2 How common is PLMD?

The prevalence of PLMD (i.e. with insomnia or hypersomnia) is not known. Around 80% of people who have RLS also have these periodic movements in sleep, but only 30% of people who have periodic limb movements have RLS. In other words, 70% of people with periodic limb movements in sleep do not have RLS. Patients with PLMD alone rarely present to sleep clinics.

Many drugs increase these periodic movements, as with RLS, and these must be assessed. They include antidepressants, stimulants (including those used to treat attention deficit/hyperactivity disorder), and alcohol.

Treatment is the same as that for RLS.

8.3 Parkinson's disease (PD)

Patients with Parkinson's disease suffer from a variety of sleep disorders that seem to be related to complex interactions between movement disorder, damage to brain areas that control sleep, and dopaminergic medications (Arnulf 2006).

The most common problem is excessive daytime sleepiness, which can affect 20–50% of patients with Parkinson's disease, and seems to be associated with greater disease severity, higher doses of levodopa, and sometimes dopamine agonists. Rarely, sudden unheralded sleep attacks can occur like those in narcolepsy, and these are more likely in patients with severe general sleepiness and frequent use of dopamine agonists. Treatment of this is difficult, but changing the dopaminergic drug regime may help. Obstructive sleep apnoea syndrome should be excluded.

Insomnia is reported in a large number of patients with Parkinson's disease, sometimes associated with nocturia or night-time incontinence, pain, or difficulty getting comfortable in bed. It can be associated with RLS or periodic limb movements (see Section 8.2), which are common in Parkinson's disease, and the majority of which are reported after the onset of the latter.

The incidence of REM sleep behaviour disorder (RBD; see Chapter 5) is high in Parkinson's disease. One study of 80 patients with Parkinson's disease who were followed up for 8 years found 5 patients at baseline and 27 patients at follow-up with RBD (Onofrj et al 2002). In this disorder there are vivid, unpleasant, and violent dreams and the loss of atonia during REM sleep, allowing violent and harmful sudden movement.

Some patients can suffer from visual hallucinations, and these have been attributed to the disturbance of dopamine in the visual system in this disorder. However, a small study (n = 10) of patients suffering from visual hallucinations revealed that all of them had RBD, and all experienced inappropriate REM periods during daytime naps associated with reported hallucinations (Arnulf et al 2000). This suggests that there is disruption of brain circuits involving REM sleep regulation.

8.4 Sleep disturbance in other medical disorders

A significant incidence of insomnia is reported in a wide range of medical disorders. Rheumatoid arthritis and other pain syndromes where there is nocturnal pain and reduced mobility give rise to frequent night-time awakenings, sometimes with subsequent daytime sleepiness. Patients with cancer who have insomnia have been shown to respond well to cognitive behavioural intervention for their insomnia (Espie et al 2008). People undergoing dialysis often have sleep problems related to scheduling of treatment. If they are dialysed at night, this can be disturbing to sleep, and if they are dialysed in the daytime, they are deprived of exercise and outside daylight, reducing their circadian rhythms.

Since poor sleep has a major impact on quality of life, it is worth asking any patient with chronic illness about their sleep, and taking seriously any problems that may affect their response to treatment.

8.5 Chronic fatigue syndrome (CFS)

There are many reports of sleep problems in patients with CFS. These include complaints of poor sleep quality, unrefreshing sleep, daytime fatigue, tiredness, and sleepiness. Only a few objective studies of sleep have been carried out, but these have shown no abnormalities of sleep structure or duration in individuals who are not depressed. However, these patients show increased time in bed, which leads to their having reduced sleep efficiency (time asleep as a percentage of time in bed).

Increased sleepiness as opposed to fatigue and tiredness has not been shown with objective testing.

8.6 Fatal familial insomnia

This is a very rare, recently reported disease that is also known as fatal progressive insomnia with dysautonomia or familial thalamic degeneration (Montagna et al 2003). It is a progressive disease that starts with sleep onset insomnia and leads within a few months to total lack of sleep and then to periods of stupor with enactment of dreams. Cognitive function is retained while the patient is conscious. There is associated autonomic overactivity and later some movement abnormalities. In the late stages of the disorder there are motor disturbances and body wasting. The disorder progresses to coma and finally death 6 to 12 months after onset.

The disease is caused by an abnormality of prion protein, as in Creutzfeld–Jacob disease. It is very rare, and is mostly familial with an autosomal dominant pattern, with 40 families known worldwide by 2011. A sporadic form of the disease was reported in 1999, and there have been approximately 24 cases so far.

Electroencephalogram (EEG) investigation shows that there is loss of the polysomnographic features of sleep, particularly slow-wave activity and sleep spindles. Postmortem studies reveal a degeneration of thalamic nuclei, and abnormalities in other brain areas less consistently.

References

Arnulf I (2006). Sleep and wakefulness disturbances in Parkinson's disease. J Neural Transm Suppl 70: 357–60.

Arnulf I, Bonnet AM, Damier P et al (2000). Hallucinations, REM sleep, and Parkinson's disease: a medical hypothesis. Neurology 55: 281–8.

Espie CA, Fleming L, Cassidy J et al (2008). Randomized controlled clinical effectiveness trial of cognitive behavior therapy compared with treatment as usual for persistent insomnia in patients with cancer. *J Clin Oncol* **26**: 4651–8.

Hening WA, Allen RP, Earley CJ, Picchietti DL, Silber MH (2004). An update on the dopaminergic treatment of restless legs syndrome and periodic limb movement disorder. *Sleep* **27**: 560–83.

Montagna P, Gambetti P, Cortelli P, Lugaresi E (2003). Familial and sporadic fatal insomnia. *Lancet Neurol* **2**: 167–76.

Onofrj M, Thomas A, D'Andreamatteo G et al (2002). Incidence of RBD and hallucination in patients affected by Parkinson's disease: 8-year follow-up. *Neurol Sci* **23 (Suppl. 2)**: S91–4.

Chapter 9

Pharmacology of sleep

Key points

- Control of sleep and waking involves a complex system of brain circuits
- The neurotransmitters involved are principally gamma-aminobutyric acid (GABA), noradrenaline, serotonin, acetylcholine, histamine, dopamine, orexin, and galanin
- Any drug that enters the brain has the potential to alter sleep

The underlying neuronal circuits and neurotransmitters involved in the sleep–wake process are the subject of intense research, and although there have been significant breakthroughs in the last few years (Saper et al 2005), there is still a great deal to discover. Much of current research is based on the discoveries of a neurologist called Constantin von Economo in the early twentieth century. He saw and described patients with sleeping sickness, now called encephalitis lethargica and thought to be of viral origin, which swept Europe and the rest of the world after the First World War and has never recurred. He was able to identify areas of the brain that showed damage at post-mortem in these patients. He described an area at the junction of the brainstem and forebrain that was damaged in the people who had been excessively sleepy. Since then, researchers have gradually established that there are ascending arousal pathways passing through this area, which involve a wide range of brainstem nuclei and neuro-transmitters, including dopamine and noradrenaline.

9.1 Brain pathways involved in sleep–wake regulation

9.1.1 Pathways that promote wakefulness

There are two main groups of these. The first group passes from the upper brainstem nuclei (locus coeruleus [LC], dorsal and median raphe nuclei [DRN and MRN], and ventral periaqueductal grey [vPAG]), receiving inputs from the tuberomammillary nucleus (TMN) of the hypothalamus and basal forebrain neurons, and then on and up to the whole cortex.

The second pathway goes from the brainstem to the thalamus, particularly to the nuclei that control the relay of sensory information to the cortex. Neurons in these pathways are active during waking (and sometimes during REM sleep), but are inactive during non-REM (NREM) sleep (see Table 9.1), and use acetylcholine as their neurotransmitter.

Table 9.1 Wakefulness pathways				
Neurotransmitter	Main nuclei	Neurons active during waking	Neurons active during NREM sleep	Neurons active during REM sleep
Pathways bypassing the thalamus				
Noradrenaline(NA)	LC	+++	+	–
Serotonin (5-hydroxytryptamine, 5HT)	DRN, MRN	+++	+	–
Dopamine (DA)	vPAG	+++	+	–
Histamine (H)	TMN	+++	+	–
Acetylcholine (Ach)	Basal forebrain	+++	–	+
Gamma-aminobutyric acid (GABA)		+++	–	?
Orexin (hypocretin)	Lateral hypothalamus	+++	–	–
Melanin-concentrating hormone (MCH)		–	–	++
Pathways to thalamus				
Acetylcholine (Ach)	LDT/PPT	+++	+	+++

9.1.2 **Pathways that promote sleep**

Von Economo also identified an area in the hypothalamus that was damaged in those patients who had prolonged insomnia rather than sleepiness. This is now thought to be the area crucial to the switch from waking to sleep, namely the ventrolateral pre-optic nucleus (VLPO). It is the primary seat of the sleep onset process, which sends inputs to all of the arousal pathways via the neurotransmitters gamma-aminobutyric acid (GABA) and galanin to damp down the arousal process and allow sleep. The VLPO can in turn be inhibited by 'arousal' systems such as noradrenaline and serotonin, and it has an indirect input from the suprachiasmatic nucleus (SCN, the clock nucleus).

How do these pathway systems relate to the drives to sleep in humans? The circadian process is strongly related to light, and light activates cells in the retina containing a pigment called melanopsin. These are relatively newly discovered cells, which project to a special set of neurons in the lateral geniculate body and then into the part of the hypothalamus involved in circadian rhythms—that is, the SCN. These cells are in fact a subset of retinal ganglion cells, and so are distinct from rods and cones; this may explain how most blind people can maintain a 24-h rhythm if the eyes are present. The SCN projects to the VLPO, via another hypothalamic area called the dorsomedial hypothalamus (DMH), and in humans this neuronal input provides a strong spur to sleep action during the hours of darkness. Of course, not all animals sleep in darkness, and there is some evidence that the DMH coordinates inputs from other centres—for example, related to feeding—to provide a different output message in those species that are nocturnally active.

Melatonin is a hormone secreted by the pineal gland during darkness, by consecutive acetylation and methylation of serotonin. Melatonin production is turned on in the dark phase by noradrenaline neurons of the sympathetic nervous system in the upper spinal cord that passes into the gland via the superior sympathetic ganglia. This release of noradrenaline acts through a beta-adrenoceptor to turn on the gene of the enzyme required to make melatonin so that its levels in the blood rise during the dark phase. Beta-blockers prevent melatonin production as they block the critical noradrenaline beta-receptor. In the daytime, the noradrenaline input to the pineal gland is suppressed by an output from the SCN, so melatonin levels are very low.

The circuits and transmitters involved in the sleep homeostatic (S) process are still unknown. The theory that there is a build-up of a sleep-promoting substance in the brain during the hours of waking is supported by good experimental evidence, but the mechanism whereby this substance may act is not yet known. Substance P, delta-sleep-inducing peptide, prostaglandins, and adenosine are some of the substances known to accumulate during waking.

9.2 Effects of drugs on sleep

Sleep and waking processes are controlled and influenced by a wide range of neuro-transmitters and brain receptors, and therefore any drug that affects these neurotransmitters or receptors will potentially alter sleep.

9.2.1 **GABA-ergic sleeping pills (hypnotics)**

Nearly all sleeping tablets act on the GABA-A-benzodiazepine receptor to enhance the action of GABA.

GABA is the most widely distributed inhibitory neurotransmitter in the brain, and it 'damps down' the excitability of neurons in all areas of the brain. Increasing GABA function causes not only sedation and sleep, but also muscle relaxation, memory impairment, and ataxia that can impair performance in skills such as driving, and increase the risk of falls, particularly in the elderly. Reduction of GABA signalling results in arousal, anxiety, restlessness, insomnia, and exaggerated reactivity.

The main type of GABA receptor in the brain, the GABA-A receptor, is a fast-acting receptor, which acts on a chloride-ion channel in neurons. When GABA binds to the GABA-A receptor, there is opening of the channel that allows more chloride ions into the neuron, making it less likely to fire.

Benzodiazepines and 'Z' drugs (zopiclone, zolpidem, and zaleplon) enhance the effects of GABA by lowering the concentration of GABA required to open the GABA-A channel. They act at a modulatory site on the GABA-A receptor that is distinct from the GABA binding site, changing the receptor complex so that GABA is more likely to cause the ion channel to open. They do not act directly to open the chloride channel, but only modulate the ability of GABA to do so, thus augmenting its inhibitory effects. Because they are indirect modulators of GABA and require its presence for their effect, the brain can, in principle, compensate for an overdose of these drugs by reducing GABA production—if there is no GABA then they will not work. It is believed that this explains the very high safety margin of these drugs in relation to older hypnotics, including alcohol.

Other psychoactive compounds, such as barbiturates, chloral hydrate, clomethiazole, and ethanol, also enhance GABA-A transmission like the benzodiazepines. However, at high concentrations they have another action that is independent of GABA—they can directly open the chloride channel. Because of this direct action on the chloride channel, these drugs have a propensity to be fatal in overdose, for if the channel is held open, the respiratory control neurons will stop firing and so death from respiratory arrest ensues.

The molecular dissection of GABA-A receptors has taken place in the past decade, and this has revealed that there are a number of different subtypes of the receptor, which have different GABA and benzodiazepine sensitivity and subserve different brain functions (Nutt 2006). In relation to sleep, the subtype that appears to be the most relevant is that containing the α1 subunit, which has large expression in the cortex and which mediates the sleep-promoting effects of benzodiazepines and the subtype-selective hypnotic drugs, especially zolpidem and zaleplon. Mice in which this subtype has been disabled ('knockouts') do not show a sleep response when these drugs are given, which demonstrates that these are the receptors which mediate the hypnotic effects of these drugs. However, although hypnotic therapeutic effects are mediated through these receptors, we do not yet know whether abnormalities of these are involved in the pathogenesis of poor sleep or insomnia.

Benzodiazepines and Z drugs are all effective hypnotics, but clinically relevant differences depend on the speed of onset and duration of action. Duration is usually defined by the half-life—that is, the amount of time it takes for half of the drug to be eliminated from the bloodstream. An ideal hypnotic drug is one that works quickly and does not cause hangover effects in the morning.

Benzodiazepines and Z drugs have similar effects on sleep, which depends on their onset and duration of action. All the fast-acting compounds reduce time to sleep onset, both subjectively and objectively with polysomnography. Depending on how long they act for, some prolong the duration of sleep and most, except for the very short-acting ones, decrease waking during sleep (see Figure 9.1).

All of these drugs increase sleep spindles and stage 2 sleep, and in high doses may decrease slow-wave sleep.

9.2.1.1 *Benzodiazepines*

These are used to treat not only sleep disorders but also anxiety, epilepsy, and muscle spasms, and as induction and amnestic agents for anaesthesia. All benzodiazepines potentiate the effects of alcohol and other central depressants, and are likely to make sleep breathing difficulties worse—for example, in obstructive sleep apnoea and chronic obstructive pulmonary disease.

Benzodiazepines enter the circulation at very different rates that are reflected in the speed of onset of action. The liver metabolizes them, and sometimes the metabolites are also active, which greatly extends the duration of drug action—for example, diazepam forms desmethyldiazepam, which has a half-life of 80 h. The main benzodiazepines that are used as hypnotics are temazepam, lormetazepam, and loprazolam. Their half-lives are shown in Table 9.2. Some other drugs are included for comparison, such as clonazepam, which is used in the treatment of some parasomnias.

Benzodiazepines have become less popular recently because of concerns about tolerance, dependence, and withdrawal, which although exaggerated by the UK media do have some basis in evidence.

Tolerance to the effects of benzodiazepine hypnotics in sleep disorders is not consistently reported, and the vast majority of studies of subjective sleep quality show that

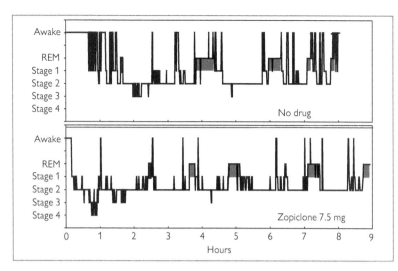

Figure 9.1 Hypnograms of an insomniac subject before and after treatment with zopiclone. Time to fall asleep is shortened, sleep (particularly stage 2 sleep), is lengthened, and awakenings are reduced throughout the night.

Table 9.2 Some properties of hypnotic drugs that affect the GABA system

	Usual dose	Rapid onset	Half-life (h)	Daytime (hangover) effects	Works selectively to enhance GABA	Safety
Zopiclone	7.5 mg	+	3.5–6	?Yes	✓	✓
Zolpidem	10 mg	++	1.5–3	No	✓	✓
Zaleplon	10 mg	++	1–2	No	✓	✓
Temazepam	20 mg		5–12	?Yes	✓	✓
Loprazolam	1 mg		5–13	?Yes	✓	✓
Lormetazepam	1 mg	+	8–10	?Yes	✓	✓
Nitrazepam	5–10 mg	+	20–48	Yes	✓	✓
Lorazepam	0.5–1 mg	+	10–20	Yes	✓	✓
Diazepam	5–10 mg	+	20–60	Yes	✓	✓
Oxazepam	15–30 mg		5–20	Yes	✓	✓
Alprazolam	0.5 mg	+	9–20	Yes	✓	✓
Clonazepam	0.5–1 mg	+	18–50	Yes	✓	✓
Chloral hydrate/cloral betaine	0.7–1 g	+	8–12	?Yes	✗	✗
Clomethiazole	192 mg	+	4–8	?Yes	✗	✗
Barbiturates		+		Yes	✗	✗
Promethazine	25 mg		7–14	?Yes	✗	✗/✓

patients report enduring effects. However, about half of the objective (EEG) studies indicate decreased effects after 4–8 weeks, implying that some tolerance develops. Dose escalation in sleep disorders is rare, and many patients claim to derive benefit with the same dose given for many years.

With regard to dependence, both animal and human research has shown that the functional characteristics of brain receptors do change in response to chronic treatment with benzodiazepines. It is thought that this is due to changes in the composition of the alpha subunits that make up the receptor; therefore they will take time to return to premedication levels after medication has been stopped. Features of withdrawal and dependence vary. Commonly there is a kind of psychological dependence based on the fact that the treatment works to reduce patients' sleep disturbance, and therefore they are unwilling to stop it. If they do stop, there can be *relapse*, where the original symptoms return. There can be a *rebound of symptoms*, particularly after stopping hypnotics, where there is a worsening of sleep disturbance for one or two nights, with longer sleep onset latency and increased waking during sleep—this is common. More rarely, there is a *longer withdrawal syndrome* that is characterized by the emergence of symptoms not previously experienced, such as shooting pains in the neck, hyperacusis, visual symptoms, altered taste, and anxiety. The syndrome is ameliorated by resuming medication, but resolves within weeks. In a very few patients it persists, and these people have been the subject of much research, mainly focusing on their personality and cognitive factors (see Figure 9.2).

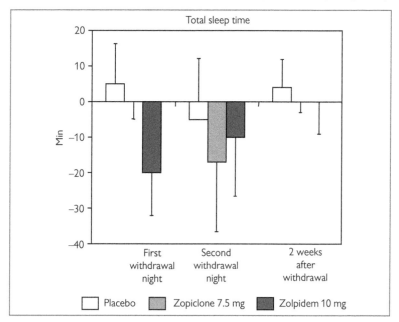

Figure 9.2 Effect of withdrawing sleeping tablets after 3 weeks of dosing in healthy volunteers. There is a rebound decrease in total sleep time one night after withdrawal of zolpidem and two nights after withdrawing zopiclone. This reflects their different pharmacokinetic properties.

Withdrawal of benzodiazepines should be gradual even after as little as 3 weeks' use, but for long-term users it should be very slow—for example, about 0.125 (1/8) of the dose every 2 weeks, aiming to complete it in 6–12 weeks. Withdrawal should be slowed if marked symptoms occur. Abandonment of the final dose may be particularly distressing. In difficult cases, withdrawal may be assisted by concomitant use of an antidepressant, dosing of which has been started a few weeks before quitting the hypnotic, so that the full therapeutic benefit of the antidepressant is present before the withdrawal symptoms appear.

9.2.1.2 Z drugs: non-benzodiazepine hypnotics that act at the GABA-A-benzodiazepine receptor

We know that these drugs act at the same site on the GABA-A receptor as benzodiazepines, because their effects are readily reversed with the benzodiazepine antagonist flumazenil. They may be associated with less tolerance and dependence, but rebound insomnia occurs after taking these drugs, as it does after taking benzodiazepines (Voderholzer *et al* 2001). Interactions with alcohol and other depressants are similar to those described earlier in this chapter for benzodiazepines, and transient withdrawal reactions occur.

- *Zopiclone*

Zopiclone is a cyclopyrrolone in structure. It has a fairly fast onset of action (about 1 h), and its duration of action is about 6–8 h, making it an effective drug for both initial and maintenance insomnia. It may cause fewer problems on withdrawal than benzodiazepines. Its duration of action is prolonged in the elderly and in patients with liver problems. About 40% of patients experience a metallic aftertaste, which is genetically determined. Some non-psychotropic drugs affect its metabolic pathway, and care should be taken to check concomitant medication. For instance, rifampicin may increase its sedative effect, and ketoconazole, erythromycin, and cimetidine reduce it, and transient withdrawal reactions occur.

- *Zolpidem*

Zolpidem is an imidazopyridine in structure, and has a fast onset (30–60 min) and short duration of action (3–4 h) (see Figure 9.3).

Patients over 80 years of age have slower clearance of this drug. It may interact with rifampicin.

Zolpidem is more selective for the receptor subtype containing the α1 subunit, and therefore may cause less muscle relaxation than is produced by other drugs in this group.

- *Zaleplon*

Zaleplon is a pyrazolopyrimidine. It has a fast onset and the shortest duration of action of the three Z drugs. Studies of psychomotor performance in volunteers have shown that it has no effect on psychomotor skills, including driving skills, when taken at least 5 h before testing (Stone *et al* 2002). This means that it can be taken during the night, either when the patient has tried getting off to sleep for a long time, or if they wake during the night and cannot get back to sleep, without a hangover effect as long as the dosing is more than 5 h before the need to drive, etc.

As with zolpidem, it is selective for α1-subunit-containing receptors.

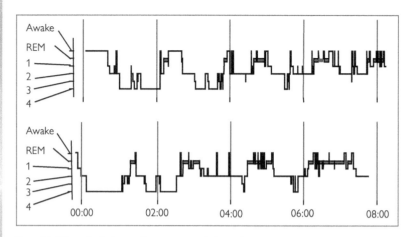

Figure 9.3 Effects of zolpidem on sleep in insomnia. In the top hypnogram, on placebo, the subject takes about 40 min to go to sleep, and has many awakenings during the night, including a long one at about 2.30 a.m. In the lower hypnogram, after zolpidem 10 mg, bedtime is earlier, sleep onset is rapid, and awakenings are reduced in the first half of the night.

- *Eszopiclone*

Recently, new chiral separation technology has allowed the active [S] enantiomer of zopiclone (eszopiclone) to be purified and used in its own right as a hypnotic. This appears to give rise to fewer hangovers than the racemic mixture that is zopiclone, perhaps because the inactive R-enantiomer has some unwanted actions. However, the most interesting aspect of eszopiclone is the fact that it has a licence for 6 months' use in the USA (not available in Europe). This is based on two placebo-controlled trials that have shown clear efficacy maintained over 6 and 12 months (Krystal *et al* 2003; Roth *et al* 2005). Although in clinical practice many patients are treated with hypnotics for many months or longer, this is the first time that controlled data showing continued efficacy and few problems during withdrawal have been available. This will be very reassuring to patients with chronic primary insomnia and their treating doctors.

9.2.2 **Other hypnotic drugs**

9.2.2.1 *Hypnotics*

Chloral hydrate, clomethiazole, and barbiturates also enhance GABA function, but are dangerous in overdose and have a propensity for abuse/misuse, so they are very much second-line treatments.

9.2.2.2 *Antihistamines*

Most proprietary (over-the-counter, OTC) sleep remedies contain antihistamines. The drug in this class with the most evidence is promethazine (not OTC), which has a slow onset (1–2 h) and long duration of action (half-life 12 h). It reduces sleep onset latency and awakenings during the night after a single dose, but there have been no studies showing enduring action. There are no controlled studies showing improvements in sleep after other antihistamines.

9.2.2.3 *Herbal preparations*

Randomized clinical trials have shown some effect of valerian in mild to moderate insomnia, but there is little evidence that it has an enduring effect (Stevinson and Ernst 2000).

9.2.2.4 *Melatonin agonists*

Melatonin is the hormone produced by the pineal gland in the hours of darkness, after a trigger from the hypothalamic nucleus (SCN) receiving input from the eyes. Early studies of melatonin were done in animals because of its effect on the oestrus cycle, and these provided evidence that administering exogenous melatonin had effects on the circadian rhythm of sleeping and waking. In the 1970s and 1980s, evidence of a drowsiness-inducing effect of melatonin in humans was found. Its use in resynchronizing circadian rhythms is now established (see Chapter 6). Melatonin and drugs that mimic its physiological action are potentially valuable compounds in the treatment of insomnia because they have no effects on motor function or balance, no hangover effects in the daytime, and no problems with rebound and withdrawal in short-term use. In the past, the findings of studies of melatonin treatment of primary insomnia have proved inconsistent (Buscemi *et al* 2005), but more recent studies with prolonged-release melatonin and with a melatonin agonist (ramelteon) are more promising.

Exogenous melatonin has a half-life of only about 1 h, whereas endogenous melatonin levels remain high during the night, and it may be that prolonged-release preparations may be more effective. Older people have lower levels of exogenous melatonin, and in two recent 3-week clinical trials with a prolonged-release preparation in older patients with insomnia, quality of sleep and morning function were improved compared with placebo (Wade *et al* 2007, Lemoine *et al* 2007). This prolonged-release melatonin is now licensed for treatment of insomnia in adults over 55 years of age.

Ramelteon, which is a high-affinity melatonin agonist at brain melatonin receptors, has been tested in primary insomnia and shown to decrease time to sleep onset and to modestly increase total sleep time after a single dose. It is licensed in the USA but will not be licensed in Europe.

9.2.2.5 *New compounds: orexin antagonists*

The wealth of new research on orexins (which are released during waking) has given rise to interest in targeting this system in the treatment of sleep disturbance. One very early study has shown that an orexin antagonist given in the daytime shortens sleep latency during a nap. More research is needed before its potential in helping night-time sleep, and its risk of inducing cataplexy, can be assessed.

9.2.3 **Antidepressant drugs**

These drugs are used not only to treat depression but also in the management of anxiety disorders. A large number of patients take them (about 28 million prescriptions are issued in one year in the UK), and therefore it is important to be aware of their effects on sleep.

Most antidepressants have profound effects on sleep architecture, particularly of REM sleep, and some also affect daytime sleepiness. Both REM effects and daytime sedation appear to be similar in depressed patients and healthy volunteers, and therefore can be thought of as markers of brain pharmacological action, but there are also effects on NREM sleep and subjective sleep, which are different in the patient population and appear to relate to therapeutic action (Wilson and Argyropoulos 2005).

The effects of antidepressants on sleep are very much associated with their effects on neurotransmitter systems in the brain, particularly their property of increasing synaptic levels of monoamines. The mechanism common to the most widely used antidepressants is that of inhibition of reuptake of serotonin (e.g. SSRIs), noradrenaline (e.g. reboxetine), and both serotonin and noradrenaline (tricyclic antidepressants and venlafaxine) into the synapse. Monoamine oxidase inhibitors (both older drugs such as phenelzine and newer, reversible drugs such as moclobemide) also increase the levels of serotonin and noradrenaline (and to a lesser extent dopamine) by preventing breakdown by the enzyme. Other drugs, such as mianserin and mirtazapine, act on the autoreceptors responsible for homeostatic maintenance of monoamine levels, blocking their negative feedback action, and so increasing synaptic levels of noradrenaline and serotonin.

As well as their main action of increasing monoamine levels, many antidepressants have (usually antagonist) effects at a variety of brain receptors, such as the cholinergic muscarinic, $\alpha 1$ and 2 adrenoceptor, histamine H1, and serotonin receptors.

9.2.3.1 *Effects on sleep architecture: selective serotonin reuptake inhibitors (SSRIs) and venlafaxine*

There are two major REM sleep effects described with all SSRIs and venlafaxine, which are dose related. These consist of reduction in the overall amount of REM sleep over the night, and a delay of the first entry into REM sleep (increased REM onset latency, or ROL), which together can be called REM suppression. This is usually obvious early in treatment, and the size of the effect is similar with all SSRIs except fluoxetine, for which the changes are generally smaller. The decrease in REM amount becomes less evident after chronic treatment, but REM onset latency remains long throughout treatment.

This REM suppression after SSRIs and venlafaxine is probably caused by the increased levels of synaptic serotonin, and it is probable that this stimulates serotonin receptors of the 5HT1A type in the brainstem REM-initiating areas, which in turn inhibits the initiation of REM sleep.

Changes in NREM sleep and sleep maintenance after acute SSRIs are also similar in volunteers and depressed patients, and consist of increased light (stage 1) sleep and waking during the night. In general, the magnitude of this arousing effect is larger in normal volunteers, but depressed patients start out with very disrupted sleep, and further deterioration is therefore less obvious. In general, these sleep disturbance effects diminish over time, with most studies in depressed patients showing no difference from baseline after a few days of treatment. The exception to this is fluoxetine, which tends to continue to disrupt sleep continuity. Fragmentation of sleep probably occurs through postsynaptic 5HT2 receptors. It can be a problem, and many doctors use a hypnotic to minimize the insomnia and distress that these drugs can induce. Recently, a study has compared the therapeutic response to fluoxetine with and without cotreatment with the new hypnotic eszopiclone. They found that depression scores improved significantly more in the group which was given the hypnotic, and that this effect was not simply due to their having better scores on the sleep items on the depression scales (Fava *et al* 2006).

The newer dual-reuptake inhibitor duloxetine has smaller effects on REM and sleep continuity than venlafaxine, despite its similar pharmacology.

9.2.3.2 *Effects on sleep architecture: tricyclic antidepressants (TCAs)*

The effects of TCAs on REM are in general similar to those of SSRIs, probably because most of these drugs increase the synaptic availability of either noradrenaline or serotonin. Clomipramine and imipramine seem to be the most REM-suppressing TCAs. The only tricyclic that does not strongly suppress sleep is trimipramine, which differs from the other TCAs in that it is only a weak uptake inhibitor.

The TCAs also differ from each other in their effects on sleep initiation and maintenance. Clomipramine, desipramine (a selective noradrenaline uptake blocker), and imipramine tend to disrupt sleep on the first night, with increased amounts of waking during sleep. After a few days, this effect is no longer present in patients, but continues in normal volunteers who were good sleepers at baseline. In contrast, amitriptyline and dosulepin improve sleep acutely in normal volunteers, but not in depressed patients. After a few days of treatment, most studies show no difference in sleep continuity from baseline. Trimipramine is remarkably sleep promoting, with decreased sleep onset latency, higher sleep efficiency, and longer sleep times reported in acute studies of normal volunteers and depressed patients. The effects may be sustained into chronic treatment in depression.

Why are there differences between drugs of the same class? The small effect of trimipramine on monoamine uptake and potent α1-adrenergic-blocking properties may explain its marked sleep-promoting effects. Trimipramine and other TCAs which are histamine H1 antagonists might be expected to reduce arousal processes, and the anticholinergic properties of TCAs might also affect arousal and sleep continuity through general arousal networks, but the sleep-promoting TCAs are no more or less active at these receptors than the other tricyclics are. There is an interesting difference in their effect at postsynaptic 5HT2 receptors; amitriptyline is a 5HT2 antagonist, and antidepressants such as trazodone and mirtazapine, and antipsychotics which are 5HT2 antagonists, such as olanzapine, are known to be sleep promoting.

9.2.3.3 *Effects on sleep architecture: monoamine oxidase inhibitors (MAOIs)*

The REM suppression after the older, reversible MAOIs is the most marked of all the antidepressants. Total suppression of REM after about a week of treatment, at doses in the range 45–75 mg/day, with the most popular MAOI, phenelzine, has been described in at least two studies of depressed patients. It appears to take longer for the REM suppression to appear than with TCAs and SSRIs. An important recent finding is that the REM suppression by phenelzine is reversed by rapid tryptophan depletion, which suggests that its REM effects occur via increased serotonin function (Landolt *et al* 2003).

In addition to these actions on REM, phenelzine and also tranylcypromine decrease total sleep time and fragment sleep both acutely and chronically, presumably because they increase serotonin and noradrenaline availability.

9.2.3.4 *Effects on sleep architecture: other antidepressants*

Mirtazapine and the related drug mianserin block α2-adrenoceptors, and therefore indirectly increase synaptic noradrenaline by reducing autoinhibition. Mirtazapine has the additional property of indirectly stimulating 5HT neurons, thus increasing synaptic serotonin. Mirtazapine has small effects on REM onset latency. It has a robust and sustained effect in improving sleep continuity in depressed patients, which is likely to be mediated by its 5HT2-receptor-blocking and histamine-receptor-antagonist actions.

Trazodone is a weak serotonin uptake blocker and a 5HT2 blocker, and also has α1-adrenoceptor-blocking effects. It improves sleep continuity in depressed patients in the same way as mirtazapine.

Agomelatine is a melatonin agonist and 5HT2 antagonist. It is reported to improve subjective sleep in depressed patients, although it has only minor effects on sleep architecture. There is also an early report of effective treatment of REM behaviour disorder (see Chapter 5) in a small group of patients (Bonakis *et al* 2012).

Reboxetine is a noradrenaline uptake blocker with no direct action on serotonergic transport. It is very selective and has little action at other brain receptors. It suppresses REM sleep with the same pattern as TCAs and SSRIs, but less markedly. It seems to have no significant effect on sleep continuity.

Bupropion is an antidepressant whose mode of action has been suggested to be uptake blockade of dopamine and noradrenaline, and it may also be a releasing agent. It too has little action at other brain receptors. Dopamine-increasing drugs do not generally have effects on REM sleep, and bupropion has no consistent effect.

Figure 9.4 summarizes the effects of different antidepressants on REM sleep.

9.2.3.5 *Subjective effects of antidepressants on sleep*

Patients and volunteers do not appear to be aware of the major effects of antidepressants on REM sleep. However, some complain of increased vividness of dreaming early in treatment, perhaps as the REM periods are delayed and the last one coincides with normal waking times.

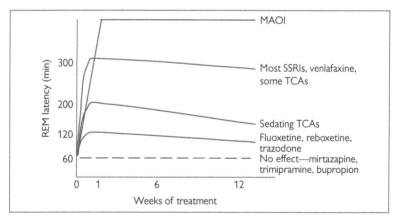

Figure 9.4 Effects of different antidepressant drugs on REM latency in depression. At baseline, REM latency is abnormally short, and this increases rapidly and markedly with the SSRIs and TCAs. The effect is slower with MAOIs, but these drugs completely abolish REM after about 1 week.

Healthy volunteers complain of poor sleep maintenance matching the disrupted sleep architecture described earlier. However, the subjective effects of these drugs in depression are complex and much influenced by the illness status. Fragmented sleep may be perceived less when mood has improved (Argyropoulos *et al* 2003). However, early in treatment, depressed patients do experience the effects of antidepressants with regard to improving or worsening sleep maintenance, and those drugs that improve it may encourage continuing compliance in people whose sleep problems are distressing.

9.2.3.6 *Daytime sedation*

Many antidepressants have effects on vigilance levels or psychomotor function that lead to impairment of performance in daytime functioning. This can have serious implications for tasks such as driving a vehicle or operating machinery. It is mainly the older drugs such as TCAs, that affect central muscarinic acetylcholine or H1 histamine receptors, which produce these effects. However, sedative side effects have been reported with nearly all antidepressants, and a wise precaution would be to warn patients at the time of first prescription not to drive until an adequate period has elapsed in which they can assess its sedative action (i.e. 1–2 weeks).

9.2.4 **Antipsychotics**

Most antipsychotic drugs affect a variety of brain receptors to varying degrees. In addition to blocking dopamine D2 receptors, they also have actions on serotonin (5HT2 receptor antagonists), noradrenaline (α1 antagonists), histamine (H1 antagonists), and muscarinic (Ach antagonists) receptors. Therefore their effects on sleep are also varied and difficult to interpret.

In the few studies that have been conducted in healthy volunteers, both older (typical) and newer (atypical) antipsychotics decrease waking during sleep. Olanzapine also increases total sleep time and slow-wave sleep, and delays REM onset.

The typical antipsychotics haloperidol and flupentixol and the atypical antipsychotics olanzapine, risperidone, and clozapine tend to decrease sleep onset latency and improve sleep maintenance in schizophrenia patients (Monti and Monti 2004).

Subjective sleep improvements have been reported after most antipsychotics, particularly chlorpromazine, risperidone, olanzapine, and quetiapine.

9.2.5 **Wakefulness-promoting drugs**

Amphetamine-like stimulants increase wakefulness by blocking dopamine reuptake, by stimulating dopamine release, or by both mechanisms. Modafinil may increase wakefulness through activation of the noradrenergic and dopaminergic systems, possibly through interaction with the orexin system. Caffeine inhibits adenosine receptors, which can in turn produce activation via interaction with GABAergic and dopaminergic neurotransmission. These drugs are detrimental to sleep, and patients who take them, and their doctors, should be careful to time the dosing so that the stimulant effects do not impinge on desired sleep.

9.2.5.1 *Caffeine*

The duration of the effects of caffeine on waking varies greatly from person to person, probably due to genetic differences in adenosine receptors, and it can also change as we get older, probably due to genetic differences in adenosine receptors. In experimental studies, caffeine produces extension of sleep onset time and modestly increased wakening at night when taken in doses of about 150 mg at bedtime (equivalent to 1 to 2 cups of brewed coffee). It may also alter the structure of sleep, delaying the slow-wave sleep peak early in sleep.

9.2.5.2 *Amphetamines and amphetamine-like drugs*

Dexamfetamine and methylphenidate are used to treat narcolepsy and other hypersomnias, and attention deficit hyperactivity disorder (ADHD), and for military purposes in some countries. Sleep architecture studies show that they increase awakening during sleep and decrease deeper sleep. Dexamfetamine reduces REM sleep and increases REM latency, and methylphenidate may do this, too, but has not been studied so extensively. There is a marked rebound in sleepiness and in REM sleep after withdrawal.

9.2.5.3 *Modafinil*

Modafinil is a wakefulness-promoting drug that was developed as an alternative to stimulant-like amphetamines for the treatment of narcolepsy. It has little effect on sleep architecture or subjective sleep in the dose regime that is used in narcolepsy. However, at the high doses used in military situations, it prevents sleep, and in recovery sleep its effects on slow-wave sleep and REM are similar to those observed after sleep deprivation without drug.

9.2.6 **Other drugs**

9.2.6.1 *Oxybate*

The new agent for treatment of cataplexy in narcolepsy, sodium oxybate, has marked and interesting effects on subjective sleep and sleep architecture.

It is the sodium salt of gamma-hydroxybutyric acid (GHB), which probably acts mainly through GABA-B receptors in the brain, but may have a neurotransmitter system of its own (GHB receptors). It may also be metabolized to GABA, so may affect GABA-A receptors, too. This drug is abused for its euphoriant, intoxicating, and growth-hormone-promoting effects. Its half-life in plasma is very short, but its central effects are somewhat longer-lasting.

Its effects on sleep are to shorten sleep latency, reduce waking, and markedly increase slow-wave sleep. In narcolepsy, it appears to reduce the fragmented occurrence of REM sleep, decreasing the episodes and lengthening them.

In narcolepsy, it is given in doses of up to 9 g per day in two doses, the first at bedtime and the second dose 2–4 h later. Its sedative effects can be apparent for about 6 h after dosing.

9.2.6.2 *Alcohol*

In healthy good sleepers who are light social drinkers, the effects of going to bed with a blood alcohol concentration (BAC) of about 0.03% (i.e. after about two drinks) on sleep architecture are small. Slow-wave sleep is increased slightly in the first half of the night and decreased in the latter half. If the BAC is 0.1% (i.e. after five or six drinks) there is a larger effect, with sleep onset latency, light stage 1 sleep and awakenings reduced, and slow-wave sleep increased in the first half of the night and decreased in the second half (Feige *et al* 2006). In this same study, subjects were recorded with alcohol for three consecutive nights and then for the next two nights without alcohol. There was no rebound effect on withdrawal, and the authors remarked that this was probably because the rebound occurred later on the drinking night.

Chronic alcoholics show a decrease in slow-wave sleep and an increase in waking during sleep in early abstinence (see Chapter 7).

9.2.6.3 *Opiates*

Sleep after oral morphine in normal subjects shows decreased slow-wave sleep, and when morphine is given intravenously there is also REM suppression. Methadone has similar effects to oral morphine, but these are less obvious (Wang and Teichtahl 2007). In early studies of opiate addicts, who were mainly prisoners, these effects of methadone were accompanied by sleep fragmentation. In our own studies of opiate addicts undergoing inpatient detoxification from methadone, sleep effects at baseline were extremely variable. Subjects were nearly all polydrug users and had taken a variety of drugs, such as crack cocaine, benzodiazepines, and on-top heroin in the days before admission, so rebound effects from these made interpretation very difficult.

During withdrawal from heroin there is major sleep disruption, with reduced total sleep and increased sleep onset latency. This resolves within 3 to 7 days. However, in studies after methadone withdrawal, insomnia appears to last for much longer and can be present 6 to 8 weeks after the last methadone dose.

9.2.6.4 *Ecstasy (3,4-methylenedioxy-N-methylamphetamine, MDMA)*

There have been no acute studies of sleep after ecstasy use. This drug is used in situations where people want to be awake, but surveys have shown that sleep is fragmented for the two nights after, say, weekend use. There has been a polysomnography study after another drug with similar effects, called Eve (3,4 methylenedioxyethamphetamine) (Gouzoulis *et al* 1992). In this study, subjects were dosed at 11 p.m. and went to sleep normally. They woke after 1–2 h and stayed awake for about 3 h. Subsequent sleep showed total REM suppression. This would be expected, as the drug releases serotonin, and increased serotonin function suppresses REM sleep.

Long-term users of ecstasy have been reported to have disrupted sleep in two studies, but not in others.

9.2.6.5 *Cannabis*

Many users report beneficial effects on sleep, which may be mediated through increased relaxation at bedtime, as there are few objective effects on sleep. In a controlled study using nasal sprays (Nicholson *et al* 2004), high doses of delta-9-tetrahydrocannabinol (Δ9-THC), one of the main constituents of cannabis, appeared to have no objectively measured effects on sleep, but increased sleepiness on awakening in the morning. The combination of high doses of both THC and cannabidiol (CBD) (the other main constituent of smoked cannabis) produced more wakefulness during sleep and less morning sleepiness.

9.2.6.6 *Antihypertensive drugs*

Beta-blockers can induce sleep fragmentation or vivid or unpleasant dreaming in some patients, perhaps because most of these drugs also affect serotonin receptors in the brain. Changes in dreaming are also seen after treatment with anticholinesterase drugs used in dementia and in myasthenia. Clonidine is another antihypertensive drug that has effects on sleep, but these are opposite to those of the beta-blockers, as clonidine improves sleep continuity and suppresses REM sleep. These actions have been utilized for the treatment of RBD (see Chapter 5), and are also helpful when clonidine is used in opiate withdrawal.

9.2.6.7 *Anticonvulsants*

Many of these drugs have global effects on brain function, so they would be expected to affect sleep. However, they have been relatively little studied, probably because the drugs themselves and the underlying disorders of epilepsy complicate interpretation of polysomnographic electroencephalogram (EEG) analysis. Carbamazepine has been shown to increase slow-wave sleep in healthy volunteers, and epileptic patients on carbamazepine have higher levels of slow-wave sleep than do controls.

9.2.7 **Withdrawal from psychotropic drugs**

As many neurotransmitters are involved in sleep and arousal processes, any drug that causes changes in neurotransmitters and has been administered for a long period has the potential to alter sleep when it is withdrawn abruptly. For instance, there may be a rebound of REM sleep after stopping antidepressants, and this is associated with more dreaming and increased vividness of dreams. Stopping sleeping tablets and other sedative drugs often results in a rebound of wakefulness with insomnia for a few nights.

References

Argyropoulos SV, Hicks JA, Nash JR *et al* (2003). Correlation of subjective and objective sleep measurements at different stages of the treatment of depression. *Psychiatry Res* **120**: 179–90.

Bonakis A, Economou NT, Papageorgiou SG, Vagiakis E, Nanas S, Paparrigopoulos T (2012). Agomelatine may improve REM sleep behavior disorder symptoms. *J Clin Psychopharmacol* **32**: 732–4.

Buscemi N, Vandermeer B, Hooton N *et al* (2005). The efficacy and safety of exogenous melatonin for primary sleep disorders. A meta-analysis. *J Gen Intern Med* **20**: 1151–8.

Fava M, McCall WV, Krystal A *et al* (2006). Eszopiclone co-administered with fluoxetine in patients with insomnia coexisting with major depressive disorder. *Biol Psychiatry* **59**: 1052–60.

Feige B, Gann H, Brueck R *et al* (2006). Effects of alcohol on polysomnographically recorded sleep in healthy subjects. *Alcohol Clin Exp Res* **30**: 1527–37.

Gouzoulis E, Steiger A, Ensslin M, Kovar A, Hermle L (1992). Sleep EEG effects of 3,4-methylenedioxyethamphetamine (MDE; "eve") in healthy volunteers. *Biol Psychiatry* **32**: 1108–17.

Krystal AD, Walsh JK, Laska E *et al* (2003). Sustained efficacy of eszopiclone over 6 months of nightly treatment: results of a randomized, double-blind, placebo-controlled study in adults with chronic insomnia. *Sleep* **26**: 793–9.

Landolt HP, Kelsoe JR, Rapaport MH, Gillin JC (2003). Rapid tryptophan depletion reverses phenelzine-induced suppression of REM sleep. *J Sleep Res* **12**: 13–18.

Lemoine P, Nir T, Laudon M, Zisapel N (2007). Prolonged-release melatonin improves sleep quality and morning alertness in insomnia patients aged 55 years and older and has no withdrawal effects. *J Sleep Res* **16**: 372–80.

Monti JM, Monti D (2004). Sleep in schizophrenia patients and the effects of antipsychotic drugs. *Sleep Med Rev* **8**: 133–48.

Nicholson AN, Turner C, Stone BM, Robson PJ (2004). Effect of delta-9-tetrahydrocannabinol and cannabidiol on nocturnal sleep and early-morning behavior in young adults. *J Clin Psychopharmacol* **24**: 305–13.

Nutt D (2006). GABAA receptors: subtypes, regional distribution, and function. *J Clin Sleep Med* **2**: S7–11.

Roth T, Walsh JK, Krystal A, Wessel T, Roehrs TA (2005). An evaluation of the efficacy and safety of eszopiclone over 12 months in patients with chronic primary insomnia. *Sleep Med* **6**: 487–95.

Saper CB, Scammell TE, Lu J (2005). Hypothalamic regulation of sleep and circadian rhythms. *Nature* **437**: 1257–63.

Stevinson C, Ernst E (2000). Valerian for insomnia: a systematic review of randomized clinical trials. *Sleep Med* **1**: 91–9.

Stone BM, Turner C, Mills SL *et al* (2002). Noise-induced sleep maintenance insomnia: hypnotic and residual effects of zaleplon. *Br J Clin Pharmacol* **53**: 196–202.

Voderholzer U, Riemann D, Hornyak M *et al* (2001). A double-blind, randomized and placebo-controlled study on the polysomnographic withdrawal effects of zopiclone, zolpidem and triazolam in healthy subjects. *Eur Arch Psychiatry Clin Neurosci* **251**: 117–23.

Wade AG, Ford I, Crawford G *et al* (2007). Efficacy of prolonged release melatonin in insomnia patients aged 55–80 years: quality of sleep and next-day alertness outcomes. *Curr Med Res Opin* **23**: 2597–605.

Wang D, Teichtahl H (2007). Opioids, sleep architecture and sleep-disordered breathing. *Sleep Med Rev* **11**: 35–46.

Wilson S, Argyropoulos S (2005). Antidepressants and sleep: a qualitative review of the literature. *Drugs* **65**: 927–47.

Chapter 10

Coping with irregular working hours: preventing sleep problems in doctors, nurses, and other health professionals

Long and irregular working hours and difficult, responsible work with limited resources are just some of the stresses experienced by doctors and other health professionals (Ahmed-Little 2007). On top of all this are often extra stressors such as sleep deprivation and fatigue. Maintaining good sleep is therefore extremely important in order to be able to do the job properly and also to be able to enjoy life outside work. Much of the information in this chapter has been mentioned elsewhere with regard to patients with sleep problems, but is just as relevant to healthy people.

10.1 Sleep is a priority

Scheduling enough time for sleep is very important, and should not be relegated to the bottom of the list when everything else has been fitted in. Good sleep is essential for health and well-being, and if we allow it to deteriorate, there is a risk that it will not normalize once the stressful or irregular work pattern has ended. We have seen many doctors and nurses as patients in the sleep clinic, whose sleep pattern never recovered properly after they stopped working shifts or on call.

We all have different sleep requirements, but in general the standard 7–8 h in bed is probably a good rule of thumb to aim for. Many people who work in the daytime for 5 days a week, with weekends off, tend to have shorter sleep in the week and catch up the sleep debt at weekends. This is fine so long as sleep is satisfactory and tiredness in the day does not become obvious before Friday evening. However, when there are irregular working hours, a certain amount of planning is needed, in order that the sleep debt is made up adequately and in time so that we function optimally every day. There are many anecdotal reports which suggest that poor sleep and consequent daytime mental fatigue are associated with errors and omissions at work, and a study in the USA found increased attention errors in junior doctors working in intensive care settings dependent on the number of hours worked per week (Lockley *et al* 2004). Recently, an international committee of experts in circadian rhythm and sleep produced some recommendations for coping with irregular work patterns in doctors (Horrocks and Pounder 2006). These apply to all of us who need to work shifts out of hours, and some of them are included in the section that follows.

Medical practice has improved in recent years so that the worst excesses of nightly on-call with the expectation of a full day's work afterwards have been abolished under European working time directives. However, even these new working practices still mean that doctors and nurses are called upon to work night shifts at least weekly, sometimes for several nights, and to work in the daytime for the rest of the week. Understanding the basic regulation of sleep can help when forming a strategy to manage the disruption of routine that these shifts cause.

10.2 **Control of sleep**

Sleep pattern is controlled by two main processes, which were described in Chapter 1. The first is circadian rhythm, a 24-h pattern of sleeping and waking that is usually synchronized with the outside world by bright light, physical activity, and routine. Innate circadian rhythm is governed by the suprachiasmatic nucleus in the hypothalamus, which sets the timing not only for sleeping and waking, but also for liver function, hormone release, digestion, and most other bodily functions. If this pattern of light and routine is changed—for example, when travelling across time zones—it takes a few days for the internal clock to synchronize with the new environment, and if we are staying in this new environment for longer than a week, it is important to take steps to synchronize as fast as possible. Similarly, people on permanent night shifts often plan their activities outside work so that their internal clock stays on the 'day-for-night' rhythm. However, for people who only work 1–3 nights a week, it is sensible *not* to try to change the circadian drive, but to maintain a regular routine while on days.

The second process is the homeostatic process (S) or recovery sleep drive, which gets stronger the longer we are awake, as it builds up a sleep debt. When these two drives are strong at the same time, usually at around 11 p.m., then we are more likely to fall asleep readily, so long as we are fairly relaxed. It is when these two drives become separated in time that we have problems getting to sleep or waking up, and this happens when working at night. The internal clock's sleep phase is at its maximum at about 04.00 a.m., but we need to be awake then, and in the daytime the internal clock is programmed for waking when the S process is making us sleepy.

The best we can do in the short periods of out-of-hours working is to minimize the sleep debt and attenuate the external cues, which strengthen the circadian process. This will not stop us feeling tired altogether, but it will help.

10.3 Establishing a sleep–wake routine during the non-night-shift period

Box 10.1 lists some useful points. Note that these points are just as relevant for improving sleep in people who do not work nights.

Make sure that your bedroom is suitable and not used for other activities such as watching TV or using the computer. It is important to associate being in bed with being asleep.

10.3.1 Regular bedtimes

During periods of 'normal' working, it is important to schedule say 8 h in bed each night, and the critical aspect of this is deciding on a regular getting-up time and sticking to it, and going to bed 8 h before that time. Most people find that sleeping on in the morning for long periods on rest days makes it less likely that they will go to sleep quickly at their normal bedtime, so on the last rest day before a day shift it is best to get up at the workday time.

10.3.2 Morning daylight

If there is any, go out and get it! During normal working, getting morning daylight is important—for example, by being outside for half an hour soon after getting up, cycling or walking to work perhaps. This provides the light cue, which strengthens the circadian clock.

10.3.3 Exercise

It is best to take exercise in the morning or late afternoon but not in the evening, because exercising after about 7 p.m. means that the rise in body temperature and increase in circulating adrenaline levels will not have recovered by bedtime and will be arousing.

10.3.4 Winding down in the evening

Excessive arousal near bedtime will delay and fragment your sleep, so late-evening activities should be relaxing and not strenuous, upsetting, or very intellectually demanding like studying.

10.3.5 Caffeine and alcohol

Caffeine keeps you awake, and as little as one cup of coffee near bedtime will make it less likely that you will go to sleep quickly, so it is probably best to stop caffeine 4 h

---

Box 10.1 Outline plan for coping with a few nightshifts a week

- Establish and maintain a sleep–wake routine on days with normal hours and on rest days in between
- Plan naps and short sleeps to minimize the sleep debt in night shift periods
- Plan catch-up sleep in rest periods
- Eat properly, take sufficient exercise, and manage light conditions where possible
- Be aware of the effects of caffeine and alcohol on sleeping and waking

before going to bed. Alcohol tends to make you sleepier at bedtime, but as the effects wear off during the last part of the night, you are more likely to have fragmented sleep.

10.4 The day before a night shift

On this day, get up at your usual time or a bit later and have your meals as usual. In the afternoon or early evening, have a nap for 2–3 h to reduce the sleep debt for later. The effects of caffeine in tea, coffee, and cola begin to occur after about 20–30 min and last for about 4 h, so these beverages can be taken in the evening.

10.5 During the shift

During the night it is very important to try to have at least one nap, for about 30–45 min. Nurses usually plan this, but it is becoming more difficult for junior doctors, because on-call rooms have disappeared in many hospitals. There is great pressure to have these facilities restored. It is a good idea to take a caffeinated drink just *before* the nap, so that by the time you wake up, the effects will be apparent, but remember that caffeine will work for 4 h, so do not take it after about 5 a.m. Your memory and concentration are likely to be impaired for a few minutes immediately after this sleep (see Chapter 1).

10.6 The day after a night shift, if you do not have to work the next night

When you go off duty in the morning, remember that your risk of having a car accident on the way home may be increased by about three times, so if you can use another form of transport, do! If possible, try not to see much daylight—for example, wear sunglasses if it is bright. Have a light meal if you wish, and then go to bed with the curtains drawn (avoid lying on the sofa if possible, bed is best because you are used to being asleep there) and sleep for about 3 h.

For the rest of the day be active, and take your meals as usual. You will probably feel the urge to go to bed early, but if so, try to keep awake until about an hour before your usual bedtime. You will then be ready to assume your usual routine the next morning.

10.7 If you have to work another night shift

The same advice about driving home applies. It is important that your bedroom remains dark, quiet, cool, and undisturbed, because now you need to sleep for 6–7 h, or sleep deprivation will impair your functioning at night. Your family or housemates should be primed about this. If you cannot sleep for very long, try to have a nap later in the day as well (see Box 10.2). Get some exercise during the late afternoon or evening as you usually do.

Sleep deprivation and alcohol have similar effects on vigilance, and together they are additive. Alcohol will therefore have more impairing effects, especially on driving and the skills you use at work.

> ## Box 10.2 If you find it difficult to **sleep during the day**
> - Buy some expandable earplugs
> - Learn some relaxation skills
> - Do not worry about sleep or try very hard to go to sleep
> - Have a planned time to resolve home/financial/family problems each day, perhaps in the early evening, and if these problems worry you when you are trying to sleep, 'refer' them to the evening session
> - If getting sufficient sleep is a serious problem, it may be necessary to ask your GP to prescribe a short-acting sleeping pill such as zolpidem or zaleplon to be taken as needed on the days between night shifts, so long as these are not more than once or twice a week

10.8 Learning and memory

It is fairly well established that learning is consolidated and improved by sleep (see Chapter 1), and this makes it even more important to sleep after you have learned some procedural skills during the night. Also, material that is studied for exams on days between night shifts may be less successfully remembered than that studied on 'normal' days.

Take sleep seriously—for your own sake and that of your patients.

References

Ahmed-Little Y. (2007). Implications of shift work for junior doctors. *BMJ* **334**:777–8.

Horrocks N, Pounder R (2006). Working the night shift: preparation, survival and recovery—a guide for junior doctors. *Clin Med* **6**: 61–7.

Lockley SW, Cronin JW, Evans EE *et al* (2004). Effect of reducing interns' weekly work hours on sleep and attentional failures. *N Engl J Med* **351**: 1829–37.

Index